ENDORSEMENTS

This book is a diary of miracles. The stories are deeply personal about real people who found healing and power through the methods used by Dr. Books. Some of these are my friends and neighbors, and I've seen the changes recorded here. I was blessed by their stories, and I believe you will be too.

—Jeff Cotter, Master of Divinity, Presbyterian Pastor

Bernice has captured (presented) examples of Dr. Books' success in her application of techniques that gently and precisely adjust and balance physical and neurological pathways resulting in dramatic improvement of academic skills, social skills, motor skills and behavior. This presentation should provide hope to many parents for their children as well as for adults.

—*Ralph Tayloe, Ed. D., UCLA. Former Professor and Administrator with the Los Angeles Community College District*

As a traditional and holistic psychiatrist, I have enjoyed collaborating with Dr. Books. She is both skilled in the use of multiple approaches and intuitive about her patients. Continuity of care is predictable and easy. She continues to search for additional ways to make things better for people.

—John M. Ackerman, MD

"House of Miracles"

"House of Miracles"

✦

Learning Problems?
There is Help
There is Hope

Changes ARE Possible

Read about the work of Dr. Phyllis Books
Extraordinary Healer

Bernice Capelle Dotz

iUniverse, Inc.
New York Lincoln Shanghai

"House of Miracles"
Learning Problems? There is Help There is Hope

iUniverse books may be ordered through booksellers or by contacting:

iUniverse
2021 Pine Lake Road, Suite 100
Lincoln, NE 68512
www.iuniverse.com
1-800-Authors (1-800-288-4677)

The information, ideas and suggestions in this book are not intended as a substitute for professional medical advice. Before following any suggestions contained in this book, you should first consult your physician. Neither the author nor the publisher shall be liable or responsible for any loss or damage allegedly arising as a consequence of your use or application of any information or suggestions in this book.

ISBN-13: 978-0-595-40915-0 (pbk)
ISBN-13: 978-0-595-85278-9 (ebk)
ISBN-10: 0-595-40915-6 (pbk)
ISBN-10: 0-595-85278-5 (ebk)

Printed in the United States of America

This book is dedicated to teachers every where who, for years, have wondered, "Why doesn't Johnny learn it? He is being taught the same as the other students."

Contents

* From the California Research Project 2001 Spring Group

** From the California Research Project 2001 Summer Group

ACKNOWLEDGEMENTS

Thanks be to:

GOD, for giving me the ability to do the things I have done in my life.

Dr. Phyllis Books, for all her hours, days, months, and years of studying to learn how our bodies function; for gently, kindly, lovingly, treating people in many different ways to improve their health and their lives.

My Editor, who insists on remaining anonymous, for all her wisdom, help, instructions and encouragement in putting this book together properly.

Patrick Meyer, Valley PC Repair, for his expert help with my computer.

Writer Friends, for help and encouragement in rewriting.

Mary Dotz, for the new lap top computer she gave me for Mother's Day.

All my children, grandchildren, other relatives and friends, for their loving kindnesses to me.

James Vande Castle, graphic artist, for design suggestions for the book covers.

Jeff Cotter, for the front cover photo of my house.

Larry R. Rankin, for the back cover photo of Dr. Phyllis Books.

Joan Trebbow, of Joanne's Photography for the back cover photo of me, Bernice Capelle Dotz.

Dr. John Gedye for the statistics and charts on the California 2001 Project.

1

MEET DOCTOR BOOKS.
Have you ever met a lady who could offer help like this?

For years people have been told, "There is nothing you can do for your learning problems or your health problems. You have to learn to live with it. You have to adjust your life style." That is no longer true for many people. Problems such as **Dyslexia are actually reversible.**

Dr. Books has studied and studied, searched and researched in the USA and abroad, traditional treatments and alternative treatments, until she has found solutions to some of these formerly unsolvable problems. Many people have experienced unbelievable improvements in their newly adjusted bodies that have lasted for years and years, adjustments to their physical, emotional and spiritual beings that help them function normally and enjoy life.

Dr. Phyllis Books is a pioneer in working with the body and its role in the learning process. She is a grandmother, teacher, doctor, and developer of Books Neural Therapy™, a structural and neurological re-patterning technique helpful for people with learning differences, ADHD, autism, dyslexia, head trauma, allergies, migraines, confusion, stress, pain, and various other chronic health problems.

She holds a Bachelor's Degree in Education from Michigan State University, a Master's Degree in Interpersonal Communication from the University of North Texas, and a Doctorate of Chiropractic from Parker College.

She has a long list of credentials and teaching experiences in the USA, Europe, and Australia. Her alma mater, Parker College, granted her the honor of "Outstanding International Alumni" for her many contributions worldwide.

Dr. Books has done extensive post-graduate work in neuroscience, family systems, psychology, neuro-associative technique, energy medicine, pediatrics, Bio-Energetics, Cranial Sacral Therapy, clinical nutrition and more.

Trained in both traditional and energetic healing and body-mind-spirit modalities, Dr. Books utilizes primary gentle, non-force chiropractic as well as Books Neural Therapy™ and adds other healing techniques where appropriate. The latest addition to her vast repertoire of healing modalities is the:

QXCI Quantum Xrroid Consciousness Interface
EPFX Electro Physiological Feedback Xrroid
SCIO Scientific Interface Operating System
QX for short is the all inclusive-computerized system that both tests and balances the body at the subtle energy level.

The use of Quantum Technology in the health of humans and animals was developed by American Professor William C. Nelson (Bill) now based in Budapest, Hungary, using space age technology.

The QX helps Dr. Books and other health practitioners assess and assist over 9000 health problems and make suggestions for life style changes in a plan for better health.

St. Francis was for animals.
Mother Theresa was for the poor.
Dr. Phyllis Books is for children.

2

DR. PHYLLIS BOOKS: EDUCATION AND EXPERIENCE or Curriculum Vitae

Education:

1971: Bachelor of Arts Degree: Michigan State University. Major, English; Minor, Education.

1977: Master of Arts Degree: University of North Texas. Major, Interpersonal Communication; Minor, Education.

1986: Doctor of Chiropractic: Parker College of Chiropractic, Dallas, Texas.

Awards:

Outstanding International Alumni, Parker College of Chiropractic, 1996

Outstanding Chemistry Student, Mountain View College, 1986

Outstanding Female Vocalist, Memorial High School, 1964

Dean's list: Mountain View College, Michigan State University

Dean's list: Parker College of Chiropractic

Honor Table: Cigna Life Insurance Co., 1977

President's Table: Cigna Life Insurance Co., 1976–80

Agency Leader: Cigna Life Insurance Co., 1977–80

Licensure/Certification:

Doctor of Chiropractic: Texas, 1986; California, 1987

Certified Advanced Instructor: Sacral Occipital Technique, 1988

Diplomate: Bio Energetic Synchronization Technique, 1986

Expert Examiner: California State Board of Chiropractic, 1992

Diplomate: American Chiropractic Board of Nutrition, 1996

Certified Clinical Nutritionist, 1996

Advanced Training:

1979–82: Human Capacities Program: Dr. Jean Houston

1993: Holotropic Breathwork: Dr. Stan Grof

1994: Hands of Light: Barbara Brennan

1988–92: Holodynamics: Dr. Vernon Woolf

1989: Pre-Cognitive Re-Education: Dr. Rick Moss

1984–92: Music and Healing; Toning: Don Campbell

1988–91: The Magic of Healing: Dr. Deepak Chopra

1982: Gestalt Synergy: Ilana Rebenfeld

1995: Body-Centered Transformation: Dr. Gay and Kathleen Hendrix

1996: Science of Consciousness: University of Arizona

1981: Paradigm Shifts in Science, Health, and Economics: Spain; Dr. Fritof Capra; Dr. Karl Pribram; Dr. R.D. Laing; Dr. Hazel Henderson; Dr. John Halifax

1987: Healing in Other Cultures: Peru

1978–86: Human Development Council: Dr. Elaine DeBeauport

1982: Therapeutic Touch: Dr. Delores Krieger

1981–95: Neural Linguistic Programming

1987–88: Neural Associative Techniques

1995: Reiki Master

1993: Learning Enhancement Advancement Program (LEAP): Dr. Charles Krebs

1998: Emotions, Quail and Consciousness: Italy

2000: Positive Emotions: University of Wisconsin

2000: Test Of Variables of Attention: Dr. Larry Greenberg

2001: Physiology of Learning: Dr. Carla Hannaford

Additional Education

1983–89: Bio Energetic Synchronization Technique

1984–92: Sacral Occipital Research Society International

1984: Parker School for Professional Success

1984: Advanced Nutrition; Certified 2001

1984–85: Motion Palpation Institute

1984–85: Gonstead Technique

1985, 2001: Acupuncture

1987: Advanced Neural Organization Technique

1987: SOT TMJ/Cranial Work

1989: Network Spinal Analysis

1996: Torque Release Technique

1996: Clinical Nutrition

1998: Neuro Emotional Technique

1999: Nambudripad's Allergy Elimination Technique

2000: Cranial Sacral Therapy

2000: Holistic Health Practice; Dr. Brimhall

2001: Pediatric Cranial Sacral Therapy

2004: Upledger: CS Somato Emotional Release

2005: Emotional Freedom Technique (EFT)

2005: Activator Technique

2005: NBCB and NTBC-Biofeedback Certification

Work Experience:

Doctor of Chiropractic 1986—Specializing in pediatrics and learning differences.
CEO and Founder: ASSISI^{TM} Foundation 1994—Dedicated to research and treatment of children worldwide, specializing in developing health and education strategies to enhance self-value and self-responsibility of all children.
Founder: Books Neural Therapy ™ 2001
Seminar Leader/Learning Consultant, 1993–
Public Relations, Parker College of Chiropractic, 1983–4
Communications Consultant, 1981–2
Financial Consultant, Connecticut General, 1977–1981
Operations Manager, NTSU Educational Foundation, 1973–6

3

JUST WHAT IS BOOKS NEURAL THERAPY™?
A combination of treatments unlike any other.

Books Neural Therapy™ is a unique, non-force, non-drug therapy developed by Dr. Phyllis Books for treating various mechanical, neurological and emotional disorders. Books Neural Therapy™ looks at the development of the whole body, not just one part.

Books Neural Therapy™ uses a multidisciplinary approach. Books Neural Therapy™ looks at structural and neurological causes of the problems.

1. A very thorough case history is taken, followed by neurological, structural, educational/cognitive testing. Each person is unique, so a plan is developed and discussed with the patient taking into account their strengths, weaknesses and goals.

2. The nervous system coordinates body movements and brain function. Gross motor skills such as running and jumping need to be in good working order before fine motor skills such as reading and handwriting can function well.

3. The body is designed and develops in a sequential order. Biology, psychology and neuroscience are making new findings and advances in neuroscience which Dr. Books studies and adds to her protocol of treatments.

4. Books Neural Therapy™ finds the communication break down in the nervous system and then readjusts the particular neurological pathways so the entire body operates with more ease, confidence and efficiency.

5. This is done with gentle, hands on, non-invasive treatment, addressing various areas of the body with a lot of emphasis on the head, eyes, ears and TMJ (jaw joint). The doctor addresses sensory input and helps upgrade the functioning and coordination of the various senses.

6. Neurological therapy as done in Books Neural Therapy™ addresses the neurobiological development of the human being. It is foundational work in that it provides often missing building blocks to a cohesive and smoothly integrated nervous system.

7. Currently there is a lot of research on the "basic brain" which Dr. Books has zeroed in on many years ago. If this hindbrain, basal ganglia, cerebellum, etc. isn't in proper working order, higher order learning will have "glitches" in it.

8. Books Neural Therapy™ is an incredibly logical and sequential series of adjustments to the brain and nervous system which affects brain function. It seems that very few people thought of addressing the neurological system in a non-invasive, natural way. Our traditional western medical model focuses on medication and invasive surgical procedures. Books Neural Therapy™ is a totally natural and non-invasive way of dealing with natural cause and effect in the brain and body.

9. Sensory integration, often performed by occupational therapists, would have some of the components of Books Neural Therapy™, since they deal with sensory input to the brain.

10. Chiropractors and Osteopaths who deal with the spine and visceral relationships, various therapists, who do cranial and sacral therapy address parts, nutritionists, neurologists, psychotherapists, all address parts of the Books Neural Therapy™ complex. **Only Books Neural Therapy™ addresses the whole variety of therapies.**

11. For brain injuries Books Neural Therapy™ starts with the very beginning and rebuilds the primitive reflexes dealing with balance centering, progressing to hearing (auditory) and visual reflexes. Books Neural Therapy™ works with one part of the body system after the other starting with the feet, the pelvic area, the spine, shoulders, neck and jaw joints on to other parts of the skull. The TMJ (jaw joint) is the counter balance to the pelvic area. The Books Neural Therapy™ practitioner will balance the pelvic area before the jaw joint or it will not hold. Many

times the eye muscles are not coordinated. This could be from a fall or trauma; or one of the four cranial nerves that deal with the eye muscles are malfunctioning. Or the sphenoid bones which form part of the eye socket might be slightly askew. In that case the eyes will have great difficulty tracking together. If the eyes are not tracking in sync or if the eye movement and auditory channels are out of sync, reading will be much slower.

12. Treatments usually consist of about 16 to 20 half hour sessions over a two to three month period. Many people from long distances fly or drive to Austin, Texas or Solvang, California and stay for four or five days. Books Neural Therapy™ is then administered 3 or 4 times a day. Once the body finally "gets" what is normal, it wants to stay there. Unless there is another trauma, corrections are still holding after five, ten or fifteen years.

13. Some people begin to feel a difference after one or two treatments. Some people are not as tuned in to their bodies and do not feel the changes until later. Sometimes the origin of these neurological problems is hereditary. Sometimes it is due to an old fall to the head or tailbone. Sometimes it is biochemical. Sometimes it is severe allergies. Each case is individual. Dr. Books gives hope where it is realistic and truthful when current evidence indicates otherwise.

14. Nutrition, life style and daily patterns are important. Allergies and nutrition are also a part of the "big picture" approach to treating focusing and behavior problems.

15. Improved reading speed and comprehension are some of the things Books Neural Therapy™ does best. **Dyslexia is actually reversible.** Many people believe it is something you have to learn to live with and compensate for. Books Neural Therapy™ by addressing the problem at neurological and developmental levels has an 85% success rate of correcting dyslexia. We work at a permanent correction.

16. Books Neural Therapy™ does no harm. In about 15% of cases nothing happens.

17. Who can benefit from Books Neural Therapy™? People with learning problems, neurological problems, (learning has a neurological component to it) brain injuries, physical coordination problems, too much

stress......in short, almost anyone can benefit from Books Neural Therapy™.

4

BERNICE CAPELLE DOTZ, 80 YEARS OF EDUCATION AND EXPERIENCE

Some of the things I have done over the past eighty years.

Education: Graduated from Winnebago Lutheran Academy, as Valedictorian with enough credits to equal an AA Degree in California. Took various College Classes. Attended many Seminars, learned from individuals who knew what I needed to learn.

I am very thankful for the many mentors in my life.

Teacher: Taught archery and handcrafts at Camp Mount Morris summer camp, 1942, 1946; taught grades 1 through 4, 1943–1944, and 3 to 5, 1944–1946 with forty to forty-six students in one room—at Trinity Lutheran School in Brillion, Wisconsin; taught forty students in grade 1, 1946–47—at Trinity Lutheran School in Sheboygan, Wisconsin, where I met my husband of forty-six years. After marrying and moving to California in 1947, took a break to raise seven children.

Taught "Sew, Knit, and Stretch®," adult education ladies and men's wear, at our store in Carpinteria, CA 1972–1973; taught a sewing class (guest of teacher) at Northridge Junior College, Northridge, CA; taught small business class 1978 (guest of teacher) at Hancock College extension class in Santa Ynez, CA; taught both adult and children's Bible classes at various times and places.

One of the special Bible classes I taught was when we lived in the part of Los Angeles called Mar Vista, between Venice and Culver City. There were a lot of children on our block. The sad thing was that there was also a lot of fighting amongst the children.

In getting acquainted with the neighbors I found that there were Catholics, Jews, Baptists, Lutherans, as well as others. I got some sheets of Old Testament Bible stories with pictures on them from our church, and invited all the children

11

to my home on Saturday mornings. I taught the Old Testament stories and emphasized that they all believed in the same God. They all believed in the same Ten Commandments, that Jesus Christ was a Jew, that they should all honor, respect, and be friends with one another. That ended the fighting. When the Jewish family moved away she invited me over and thanked me. She gave me a lovely delicate Chinese tea set, which I treasured and which one of my daughters now enjoys in her home.

Retail Manager: For thirty-two years, sold clothing, shoes, accessories, jewelry, sewing machines. Grew sales from $150,000, per year to $500,000 per year at one small store.

Recruiting: Selected, hired, directed, trained employees, six of whom we helped to open their own stores. Older ladies stayed with us until retirement. Younger employees used our training as stepping stones to something better.

Management: While managing the primary stores, we also owned and operated a motel, wholesale nursery, wholesale ceramics manufacturing, and retail sewing machine store.

Financial Officer: We handled the financing to build eight homes. My five years of experience in banking was very helpful in this and other endeavors.

Producer: Wrote proposals, contracts, news releases, television and radio scripts.

Successfully completed two lot splits, two conditional use permits and one city ordinance.

Community Service: I was instrumental in starting the Bethania Pre-School and After-School Program, Shepherd of the Valley Pre-School, and the Solvang Farmers Market.

Started Neighborhood Day, the first Sunday of each October, beginning in 2000.

Earned Awards: Named "Woman of the Year" by the Santa Ynez Valley News and the Santa Ynez Valley Foundation, 1999. Named "Volunteer of the Year 1999" by the Solvang Chamber of Commerce; named "Business Person of the Year 1998–1999" by the Santa Ynez Valley Rotary Club. Named "Officer of the Year" by Lutheran Brotherhood. Branch 8306, February 2001. Honored by the Santa Barbara County Human Relations Commission for 2000, Third Supervisorial District.

Travel: Traveled to all fifty states and thirty-six foreign countries.

Continuing Education: My seven older brothers and sisters taught me many practical and useful things.

My oldest sister Orma (twenty years my senior) and her husband Adolph taught me how to drive a pickup truck, a tractor, and a team of horses, how to milk a cow by hand and to mow hay, how to feed the chickens and gather eggs, how to fish for bullheads, how to work hard, have fun and be healthy, without running water or electricity.

My sister Dorothy (eighteen years my senior) and her husband Joe taught me how to crochet, upholster furniture, cut glass, enjoy museums, travel on street cars, and a bit about metals and manufacturing.

My brother Carl the barber (fifteen years my senior), taught me how to cut my dad's hair because gasoline was rationed during World War II and he couldn't make the trip home often enough to do it. He also taught me how to hunt deer with a bow and arrow. He also insisted on proper English when I worked in his barbershop.

My brother Vic (thirteen years my senior) taught me how to start seeds in a hot house and transplant the delicate seedlings into flats in winter to get an early start on summer plants. He also taught me how to get involved in politics. He was elected Mayor of Fond du Lac, Wisconsin.

My brother Ira (ten years my senior) taught me how to be a teacher by babysitting his three oldest children. He taught me to dream big impossible dreams and work to make them come true.

My brother Earl (eight years my senior) taught me the value of perseverance and keeping on toward my goals.

My brother Bim (six years my senior) taught me how to love (not sexual love, but brotherly love), and laugh and have fun. He made my first bow and set of arrows and taught me how to shoot them and become Junior Girls State Champion.

To me the greatest gift parents can give their children is the gift of loving brothers and sisters.

5

INTRODUCTION: Did you ever have a chance meeting THAT CHANGED YOUR LIFE? I DID.

One of the definitions the Oxford Dictionary gives for a miracle is "a highly improbable or extraordinary event, development, or accomplishment that brings very welcome consequences". It is this description that led me to call my house the "House of Miracles". Dozens and dozens of extraordinary accomplishments took place in my home at the hands of Dr. Phyllis Books.

For more than fifty years, as a former teacher, I wondered why some children just didn't learn what I was teaching; I taught the same thing to every student in the class but, occasionally, one of them just did not understand what was going on. I hated to hold these children back, but I knew they would struggle through the higher grades if they did not have a proper foundation.

I tried various teaching techniques—phonics helped some, one-on-one teaching helped others—but some students just couldn't seem to comprehend the lessons.

I met Dr. Books at her parents' golden wedding celebration. She had come from Texas to Solvang, California, "The Danish Capital of America" for the happy occasion. In our conversation she told me that she worked with people who were "learning disabled," or as she described it, people who have "learning differences".

Dr. Books explained that some children have a neurological dysfunction that cannot be overcome by standard teaching methods. Since one of my grandsons had to repeat second grade in elementary school, and was getting D's and F's in junior high, I was very interested in the technique she developed, Books Neural Therapy™, to help these people. Since she had to fly back to Texas and could not stay to see him, she told me of a chiropractor in Santa Barbara, California (much closer to me than Texas), who did some of the alternative therapies Dr. Books does. We took my grandson to this doctor. He improved a little, but discontinued his treatments too soon.

Several months later, when Dr. Books was in town again she asked how Rick was doing. I told her he had improved a little and she said he should be doing much better than that and offered to treat him if we could get him to Solvang. Dr. Books treated him and the results were so amazing I offered her my home as a second treatment office whenever she came to California.

Mine is a humble home on a street so quiet that, when the seventy-foot-tall Eucalyptus tree in front of my house is in blossom, you can hear bees buzzing about their business. For the next several years the things that happened at my house seemed like a miracle to me. Patients shuffled to my door looking down at the ground, shoulders stooped, demeanors unhappy and skeptical. They had already tried everything anyone suggested to make a difference in their lives, but nothing helped. They worried, "Why don't people understand that I'm doing my best, but I just can't get anywhere?"

Dr. Books' gentle touch on the key spots of a body produces miracles of healing, just as her gentle touch on the keys of a piano produces beautiful music. I watched, day after day, as both children and adults, after one or more treatments from Dr. Books, left my house walking confidently, smiling, heads held high, ready to challenge the world. Imagine the joy of a child who suddenly realizes, "I can do it! I can read!" Or the delight of the lady who said, "My head doesn't ache anymore".

I was very excited and very naïve. I thought every one could be helped that quickly. NOT SO! Over the years I've learned that it takes from sixteen to twenty half-hour treatments for the average learning disabled person to improve to near grade level, with further improvements coming over time and with teaching. The variant can range from one or two treatments for minor problems to several years of treatments for major problems.

"What can I do to help spread the word about this wonderful breakthrough that helps people with learning differences?" was the question that plagued me.

This book is the answer. It tells about some of those boys and girls, men and women whose results were, to me, miraculous.

It includes a report on the research project we did in 2001.

The names have been changed to protect the privacy of the patients in this book.

Statistics vary indicating that any where from 60% to 90% of the people in jail can not read well enough to hold a good job. Wouldn't it be great if we could cut those numbers in half by using Books Neural Therapy™ to adjust their bodies so they could be successful?

Dr. Books has helped thousands worldwide through her own practice and through other professionals she has taught. For more information about what she is doing now visit her web-site: www.BooksNeuralTherapy.com or www.BooksFamilyHealthCenter.com.

Get ready for an experience that will offer you the opportunity to find help and hope for any of you who has a friend or relative with a "learning difference".

6

CALIFORNIA RESEARCH PROJECT—2001, have you ever seen students advance three grades in three months? It has happened.

Twenty four students, ages 7–20 were selected at random from Santa Barbara County in California, to participate in a study measuring the positive changes utilizing Books Neural Therapy™, a non-drug intervention to improve academic skills and social behavior. Funding was made possible through the Schlinger Foundation.

Dr. Phyllis Books did all of the treatments on these patients. I, Bernice Capelle Dotz, did most of the pre and post testing. A teacher from the "Family School", Joanne Kresse, did some of the testing on the younger students. Dr. John Gedye from Michigan did the statistics for us.

Twelve students were pre-tested with the Wide Range Achievement Test, treated with Books Neural Therapy™ for nine hours over a six week period, and nine were post tested with the Wide Range Achievement Test during the spring of 2001. Three members of one family were unable to complete the post testing.

The Wide Range Achievement Test is a commonly used quick assessment of overall reading, math and spelling proficiency. The Books Neural Therapy™ is a neurologically based, hands-on repatterning technique to improve brain integration and body function.

Of the subjects in the first group, three had been at Los Prietos Boys Camp (a detention facility in the mountains for boys who had been in minor trouble with the law).

One boy went from reading at grade four to grade twelve. The second boy, who had been to Los Prietos twice, improved three grade levels in reading, two grade levels in math and five grade levels in spelling. The third boy was one of the three people who did not complete the post testing.

The average improvement in reading for the first group of nine was three grade levels in six weeks (16.09% change in the raw scores), two grade levels in math (16.55% change in the raw scores) and unsubstantial overall changes in spelling (0.81% change in the raw scores).

Interesting to note, in the first group is the consistent improvement in both math and reading, very different skills. One of the most ADD children in this group, aged 8, made little change in reading, (he was already at grade level), but improved two grade levels in math, an unusual and very hopeful change for a creative child. Often very right-brained, artistic children don't do as well in math, a left brained activity.

The second group of twelve students were pre-tested with the Wide Range Achievement Test, The Bruininks-Oseretsky Test of Motor Proficiency, and the T. O. V. A. a computerized Test Of Variables of Attention. They were then treated with Books Neural Therapy™ and post tested with the same instruments as were utilized in the pre-test. This second group was tested and treated during the summer of 2001.

The Bruininks-Oseretsky Test measures gross and fine motor skills, such as running speed and agility, balance, bilateral coordination, response speed, and visual-motor control. Developmentally, gross motor skills precede fine motor skills. Both gross and fine motor skills in the body precede academic skills. An uncoordinated child often has neurological "glitches" which will affect his ease and speed of learning in school as well.

In this second group of children, one of the most remarkable changes, was in the Bruininks-Oseretsky Test, in which ALL children improved substantially. The average change in the raw scores was + 15.89%.

Since motor function is a precursor to improved brain integration, it was encouraging to get reports back from the parents and teachers of the leaps forward in academic skills during the following school year, following the vast improvement in motor proficiency as shown in the Bruininks-Oseretsky Test.

The Test Of Variables of Attention (T.O.V.A.) is a rather tedious twenty two minute computerized test to elicit information about visual and auditory distraction and attention, yielding valuable information for medical doctors and others who need to measure Attention Deficit Disorder with and without Hyperactivity. (ADD/ADHD). It measures neurological deficits and can be administered repeatedly (and is by medical doctors who utilize this test to determine the amounts of medication to prescribe to quell ADD characteristics).

Most remarkable, was the change in the ADHD scores of the Test Of Variables of Attention (T. O. V. A.) where there was an average improvement of 19.42%. Since this test measures underlying neurological deficits, and none of these children were on any medication during the study, this change, as well as the Bruininks-Oseretsky Test shows the Neurological improvement possible with Books Neural Therapy™.

Most experts agree that learning differences and Attention Deficit Disorder have a strong neurological component. However, Ritalin™ and other class two drugs have been the standard treatment for the neurological component. One of the goals of this study was to demonstrate statistically the efficacy of the treatments of Books Neural Therapy™, a non-drug intervention for improvement in academic skills and social behavior.

The Wide Range Achievement Test on the second group did not yield very substantial changes, probably because the preponderance of the subjects had only completed first grade and were getting ready to enter second grade, leaving little possibility for several levels of improvement.

If a child has turned off both sides of his brain, (logic and creative) due to constant frustration in school, has been labeled "klutzy" or is accident prone, has had head injuries, has structural misalignments (jaws, hips, un-level eyes), low self esteem, inconsistent behavior and performance; Books Neural Therapy™ offers a comprehensive, non-invasive, one on one, whole body-brain reintegration which improves the quality of life in general, and academic and social skills in particular.

California Research Project 2001 Spring Group Key:

	Name	Age	Gender	Education	
1	AC	10	M	4	
2	JC	14	M	8	
3	AK	8	M	2	
4	PS	10	M	4	Special_Ed
5	MS	12	M	6	
6	JV	14	M	9	
7	CV	16	M	10	Special_Ed
8	LV	14	M	8	
9	MI	20	M		

Figure 1—Wide Range Achievement Test (reading)
Spring Group 2001

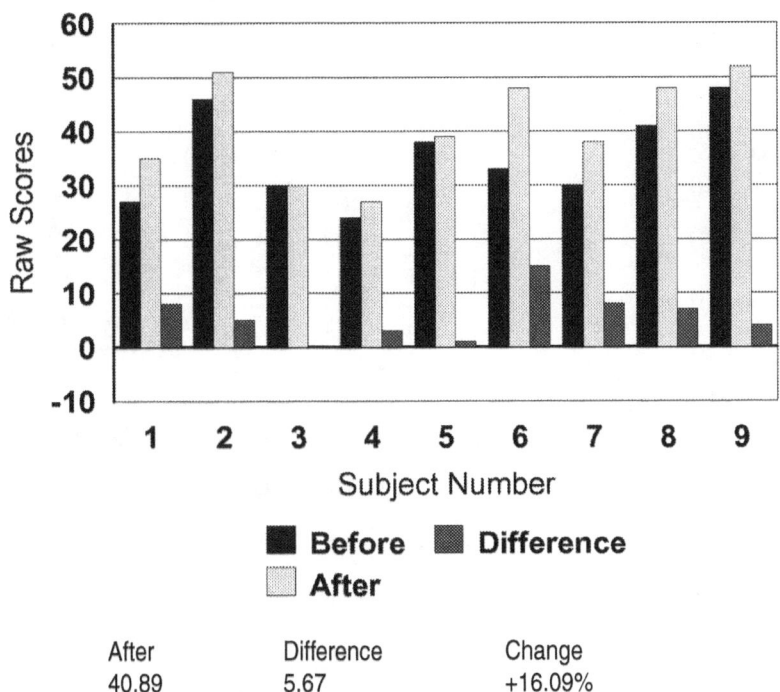

Before	After	Difference	Change
35.22	40.89	5.67	+16.09%

Wilcoxon Matched-Pairs Signed Ranks Test
$T = 0$; $N = 9$; $Z = -2.67$; $P = 0.0038$ (one-tail)**

Figure 2—Wide Range Achievement Test (spelling)
Spring Group 2001

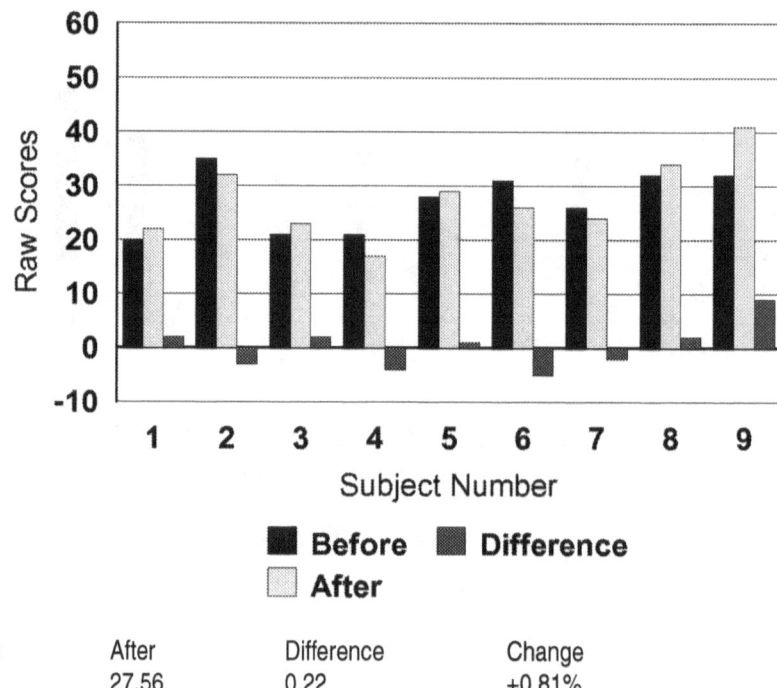

Before	After	Difference	Change
27.33	27.56	0.22	+0.81%

Wilcoxon Matched-Pairs Signed Ranks Test
$T = 24.5$; $N = 9$; $Z = 0.24$; $P = 0.4052$ (one-tail) NS

Figure 3—Wide Range Achievement Test (arithmetic) Spring Group 2001

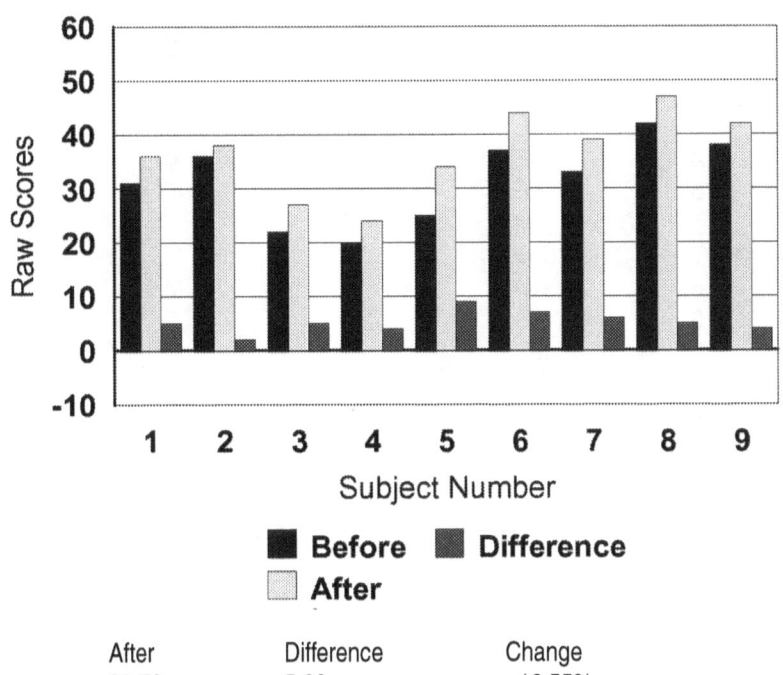

Before	After	Difference	Change
31.56	36.78	5.22	+16.55%

Wilcoxon Matched-Pairs Signed Ranks Test
T = 0; N = 9; Z = -2.67; P = 0.0038 (one-tail)**

California Research Project 2001 Summer Group Key:

Subject	Name	Age	Gender
1	SB	8	F
2	JC	8	F
3	JE	12	F
4	CE	10	M
5	KE	8	F
6	KM	8	F
7	BO	7	M
8	GO	8	M
9	KS	8	F
10	MS	12	M
11	CW	8	M
12	JY	15	M

Figure 4—Test of Motor Proficiency (Bruininks-Oseretsky) 2001 Summer Group

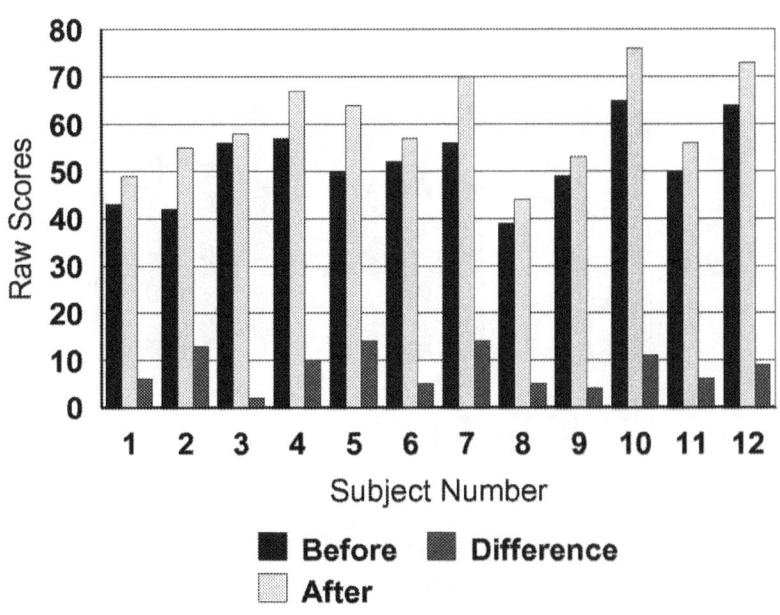

Before ■ **Difference**
□ **After**

Test of Motor Proficiency (Bruininks-Oseretsky)

Before	After	Difference	Change
51.92	60.17	8.25	+15.89%

Wilcoxon Matched-Pairs Signed Ranks Test
$T = 0$; $N = 12$; $Z = -3.06$; $P = 0.0011$ (one-tail)**

Figure 5—T.O.V.A (Test of Variables of Attention)
Visual Scores 2001 Summer Group

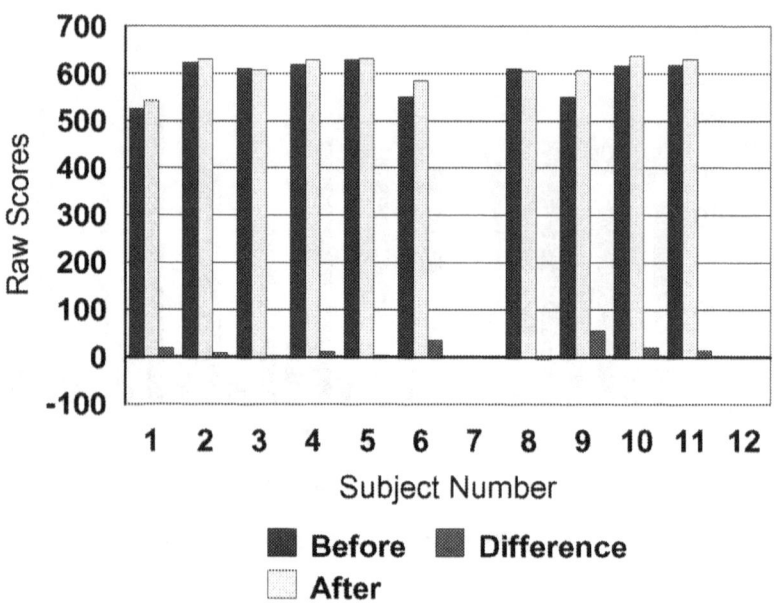

Visual Scores

Before	After	Difference	Change
592.56	608.67	16.11	+2.72%

Wilcoxon Matched-Pairs Signed Ranks Test
$T = 4$; $N = 9$; $Z = -2.19$; $P = 0.0143$ (one-tail)*

Figure 6—T.O.V.A (Test of Variables of Attention) ADHD Scores 2001 Summer Group

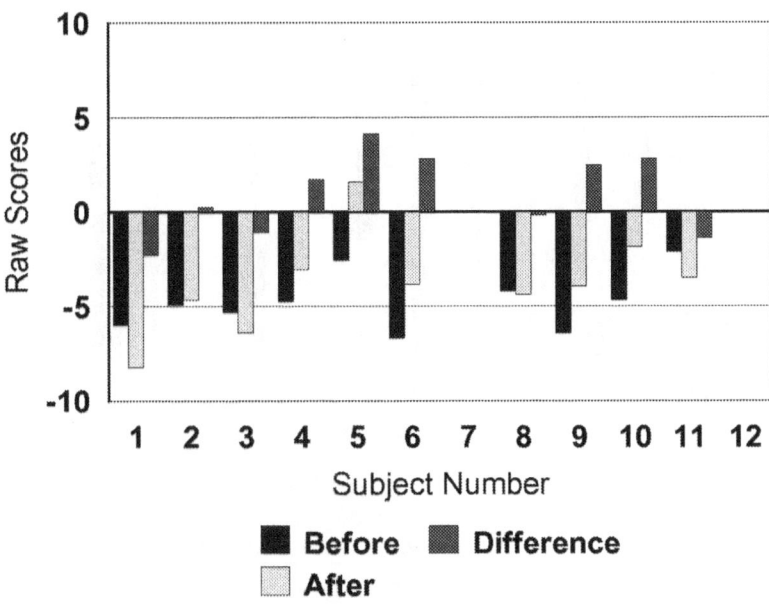

ADHD Scores (Normal range is -1.00 to +1.00)

Before	After	Difference	Change
-4.76	-3.84	0.93	+19.42%

Wilcoxon Matched-Pairs Signed Ranks Test
T = 14; N = 10; Z = -1.38; P = 0.0838 (one-tail) NS

**Figure 7—T.O.V.A (Test of Variables of Attention)
Auditory Scores 2001 Summer Group**

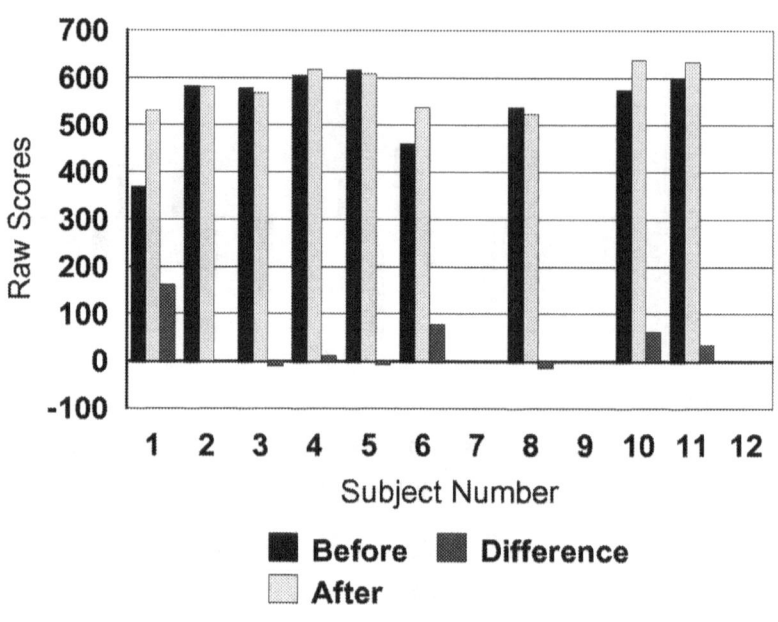

Auditory Scores

Before	After	Difference	Change
546.56	581.56	35.00	+6.40%

Wilcoxon Matched-Pairs Signed Ranks Test
T = 11; N = 9; Z = -1.36; P = 0.0869 (one-tail) NS

California Research Project 2001 Summer Group
Key:

Subject	Name	Age	Gender
1	SB	8	F
2	JC	8	F
3	JE	12	F
4	CE	10	M
5	KE	8	F
6	KM	8	F
7	BO	7	M
8	GO	8	M
9	KS	8	F
10	MS	12	M
11	CW	8	M
12	JY	15	M

**Figure 8—Wide Range Achievement Test (reading)
2001 Summer Group**

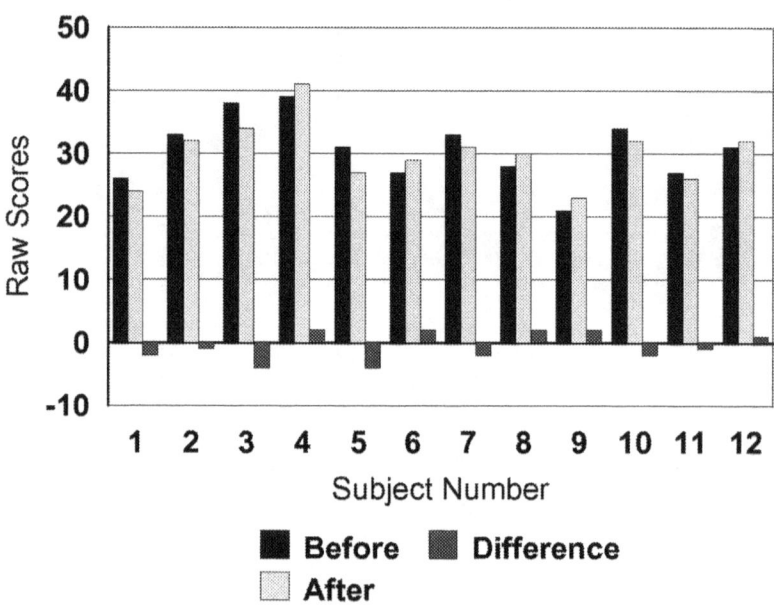

Wide Range Achievement Test (reading)

Before	After	Difference	Change
30.67	30.08	-0.58	-1.90%

Wilcoxon Matched-Pairs Signed Ranks Test
T = 42; N = 12; Z = 0.24; P = 0.4052 (one-tail) NS

Figure 9—Wide Range Achievement Test (spelling)
2001 Summer Group

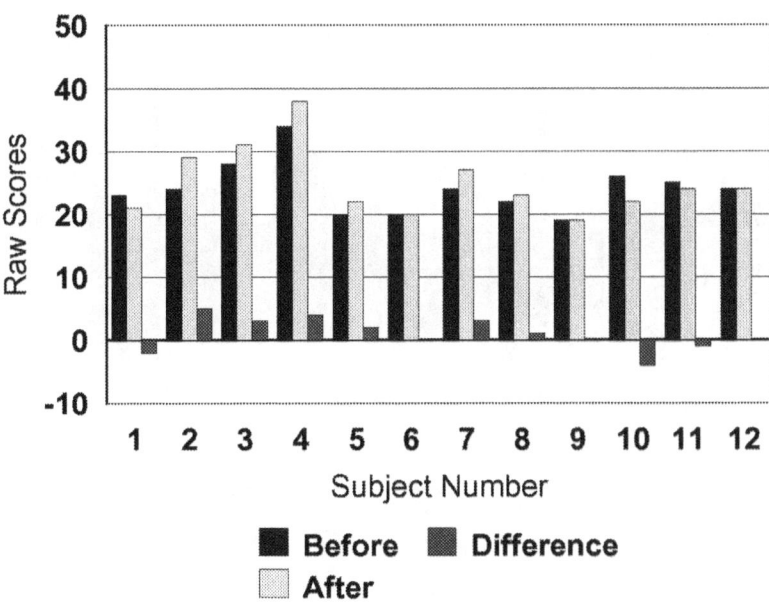

Wide Range Achievement Test (spelling)

Before	After	Difference	Change
24.08	25.20	0.92	+3.81%

Wilcoxon Matched-Pairs Signed Ranks Test
T = 12.5; N = 9; Z = -1.18; P = 0.1190 (one-tail) NS

Figure 10—Wide Range Achievement Test (arithmetic) 2001 Summer Group

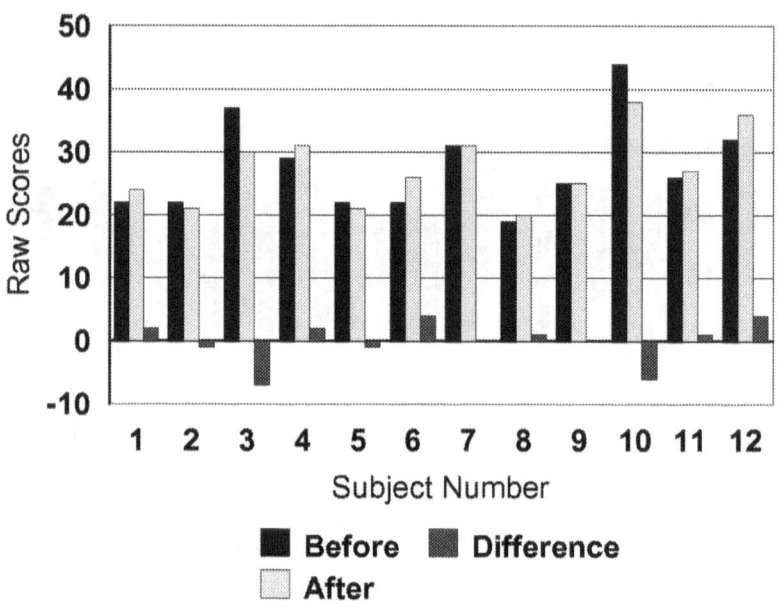

Wide Range Achievement Test (arithmetic)

Before	After	Difference	Change
27.58	25.44	-0.08	-0.30%

Wilcoxon Matched-Pairs Signed Ranks Test
$T = 37; N = 10; Z = 0.97; P = 0.1660$ (one-tail) NS

7

WERE YOU EVER AMAZED WHEN YOU SAW SOME UNBELIEVABLE RESULTS?
I was when I saw the results of Dr. Books work on Rick.

One of my grandsons, Rick, had repeated second grade in elementary school and was getting D's and F's in junior high. When I met Dr. Books and learned about her work I told her about Rick and his problems. Then I inquired about the possibility of Rick getting similar treatments locally. I found a chiropractor in Santa Barbara, California, who does some of the alternative therapies Dr. Books does.

Several months later, when Dr. Books returned to Solvang to visit her parents, I accidentally met them at a local restaurant. During our conversation she inquired about Rick, I explained his progress and she responded, "He should be doing much better than that. If you can get him to Solvang, I'll work on him".

I contacted Rick's family in Santa Barbara, and he was brought to Solvang. We met at Dr. Books' parents' home. While Dr. Books' mother, Rick's mother, and I watched, Dr. Books began treating Rick. First she had him read aloud. He…read…like…this from the *Reader's Digest*. When she asked him to walk down the hall we saw that he was a little pigeon-toed. She measured his height and then had him lie down on the portable treatment table. Starting with his feet and legs she showed us that one of his legs was shorter than the other. She evened them out. Moving up his body she found that he was having problems with his hips, spine, neck, skull, jaw joints, and the muscles around his eyes. All of these physical asymmetries were affecting his ability to learn, according to her. She proceeded to explain to us what she was doing as she balanced Rick's body.

Gently and carefully she began addressing his muscles and bones, bringing them into alignment. She worked very slowly, very carefully, using gentle pressure on just the right spots.

When she finished, Rick walked straight down the hall without turning in his toes. He read from the magazine again and read fluently. He was three-quarters of an inch taller when she finished the treatments. What she did in that one afternoon usually takes her sixteen to twenty treatments over a period of days or weeks. It helped that Rick had had a few previous treatments from the other doctor. It seemed like a miracle to me that such improvements were even possible.

In high school Rick started getting A's and B's. School work was easier for him. Reading was more endurable. His self confidence improved. He also got a part time job.

After high school Rick followed his dream and went to Arizona to a technical school and became a certified Auto Mechanic.

Having completed his 18 month auto mechanic training, Rick returned to the Central Coast of California and is now working as an Auto Mechanic. I spoke with him recently. He said he was doing fine and didn't feel a need for any further treatments.

8

CAN A PERSON HAVE DYSLEXIA AND STILL BE AN ARTIST? FLOYD had the possibility inside him.

When Dr. Books began coming to Solvang, I invited a number of friends to my house one evening to get acquainted with her and her work. Among these friends was a lady whose ex-husband is a prominent sculptor. She was concerned about her stepson, Floyd. Floyd's mother and stepmother had become friends and allies in the raising of all three sons. When his stepmother heard Dr. Books speak at my house she realized that "Books Neural Therapy™" was what Floyd needed. My friend was therefore eager to share the news about Dr. Books' work with Floyd's mother.

Floyd's father and mother agreed, and Floyd came to my house for treatments. In exchange, Dr. Books would receive one of Floyd's father's beautiful sculptures.

Floyd's mother was very ill all during her pregnancy with Floyd. The contractions were hard and one minute apart the entire nineteen hours before Floyd was born, and, in her words, the baby was "crusty and blue and green and very sick".

Floyd did not crawl or talk until he was a year and a half old. He stuttered when he started to talk. When he was about four or five he would draw very intricate designs, far more complex than the average preschooler. But by the age of seven he put away his crayons and ink, his spirit thoroughly squelched by unkind remarks from teachers and classmates.

All his life Floyd suffered with allergies that made it difficult to concentrate. Sometimes he felt dizzy. Floyd said that sometimes his head would pound so hard it felt like a herd of horses was running through it. This pressure, which had

35

developed during the birth process, had never been relieved. This, of course, caused learning problems. He loved outdoor physical activities like riding motorcycles, snowboarding, and surfing, but mental activities in school were very difficult.

Floyd's mother had become very frustrated with the school system because her son was not learning to read. He had difficulty following instructions, and when he tried to read he would reverse the letters, a sign of **dyslexia**. He could not remember to turn in his homework, would trip over his words when he tried to talk, and had a hard time finishing his work. One day he would be able to perform a particular task and the next day he could not. It was not because the teachers were not trying, or the parents were not cooperating, or Floyd was not working at it, it was because he had some kinks in his neurological hoses so that the messages he saw with his eyes did not process in his brain. This was very frustrating to him. He often wanted to drop out of school.

Another problem Floyd had was confusing left and right, a skill necessary for following directions to a destination.

After the initial series of treatments, when it was time for Floyd to read aloud, Dr. Books called his mother and me into the room to listen. When his mother, with tears in her eyes, heard him read, she said, "This isn't my child! I've never heard him read a whole sentence! I've spent his whole life trying to get him to read!" Floyd was fifteen years old at this time, so the mother had years and years of effort behind her heartfelt words.

When Floyd got home about eight o'clock on Wednesday evening, his mother excitedly told his father that Floyd could read. "Yeah, right," he replied. Then for the next hour, members of the family tossed him magazines and books. He read them all. He simply and plainly read them, without stumbling or hesitation.

His mother was so excited she was calling people until midnight. The next morning at nine o'clock she called Dr. Books and asked if she would speak to the whole town on the following Sunday night. She invited not only all her friends in their small town, but also all the teachers and educators who had ever worked with Floyd—including both the County Superintendent and the local Superintendent of schools. There was standing room only at the café where they convened. Floyd's mother, stepmother, and father described to the group how Floyd had always been too shy to speak and how they had tried every system they were told about in hopes that Floyd could be helped. Nothing did much good.

Dr. Books explained that learning is not just from the neck up, it is from the whole body. The body has to be in balance. The person has to have a good foundation on their feet and be secure in their walk, with balanced legs, even hips and shoulders, and balance in their head and face. "Form and function" is important in anatomy and physiology, not just for beauty to look at but also for functioning at our best. When we are out of alignment, especially in the skull bones, learning becomes very labored and inefficient. Getting his head and facial bones balanced even made Floyd a more handsome young man.

When Dr. Books returned the next month to our town, Floyd again came in for more sessions. Miracles had continued in her absence. His skin, once an almost fish-belly white, was now pink and glowing. His muscle tone had improved dramatically. During the treatment when Dr. Books was releasing the birth trauma, she turned to the sculptor-father and asked, "If this face were a sculpture, would you consider it finished?" She pointed out the asymmetries around the eyes, the jaw and the lips.

Once the famous Michelangelo was asked how he could create the magnificent sculpture of David. He replied, "I saw David in there and simply carved away that which wasn't David". Likewise, Dr. Books removed the obstacles that kept Floyd from being the entire person he was meant to be.

At the age of fifteen, after Dr. Books had treated him, Floyd once again picked up his drawing pen. Soon, however, he changed to a chisel and followed in his father's footsteps and began sculpting. At his first art show he sold all of his sculptures; before long he had sold enough artwork to buy himself a pickup truck and a piece of heavy equipment. Now, in addition to his artwork, sculpting with serpentine stone from his father's land, he does roadwork on private properties.

9

Do you know a family that was severely damaged by alcoholism and divorce? This family was.

This young lady was charming, outgoing, had a pleasant smile, and was great with the customers. She started working at our store as a teenager. After college she took a job on a cruise line, sailing up and down the Alaskan Coast in the summer and up and down the Mexican Pacific Coast in the winter. It was fun for a few years. Then she came back home and worked at our store again.

Shortly after returning she met a handsome, talented young man, fell in love and got married.

They rented the apartment above our store, and lived there until their first baby started to crawl. Then they moved to Buellton. Over the years they were blessed with three lovely daughters.

Social drinking changed to drinking to the point of passing out regularly. This brilliant computer engineer changed. No longer the loving husband and father, he was now controlled by alcoholism. Divorce followed. He moved home to live with his mother. This addiction escalated to the point of violence.

When Sunny took the girls to visit their grandma, the girls were hoping to see their dad. They still loved their dad very deeply. Grandma told them that their dad had broken her nose when he was drunk, and she made him leave. The girls were devastated.

The years followed with no physical, written, or financial contact between father and daughters. Two or three times in ten years the dad called and promised to visit the girls, but he never showed up. The girls were so eager to see him they even went to visit the homeless shelters and talked to people who knew him, but they never found him. An investigator revealed that he had been moving from homeless shelter to homeless shelter.

The girls had a few neurological/learning issues before the divorce. Sunny believes that Dr. Books' treatments, even in the light of the emotional trauma, facilitated the eventual healing. The treatments were able to help the family in their struggle to get back to normal, but the emotional drain of the divorce and loosing their dad was devastating on the girls.

Divorce is a serious emotional trauma and one not easily treated. Books Neural Therapy™ can help with the physical, neurological and emotional trauma that happens in the body from such a devastating emotional event. With Dr. Books' treatments, time, patience and love from their friends and family the girls have recovered.

Charter school was a big help for the girls. They could be successful in that setting.

The two older girls each took a year abroad in their schooling. One went to Russia and one went to Denmark. They enjoyed and grew and matured with the opportunity to live for a year with an intact family. Both girls are now in College and have part time jobs. The younger girl is in charter high school and also has a part time job.

Dr. Books' work with this family, treating mother and all three daughters was a help through the difficult times. But no treatment can take the place of a lost father.

10

Does someone you know STUTTTER or have trouble pronouncing their words? BLAIR did.

How would *you* feel if, when you tried to speak to someone, the words would not come out, except in a s-s-s-stutter? When you tried to speak words with s's, t's, and r's people would respond, "What did you say?"

You would probably do as Blair did and avoid talking with people. You would hang your head and hope no one would speak to you. Some people would think you were rude, or shy. So, rather than be embarrassed by having to repeat what you said because it didn't come out right the first time, or the second time, or the third time you just wouldn't talk.

Blair was eight years old, going on nine, when I spoke with his mother and told her about Dr. Books' work. I had known his mother for years. She brought her family of two boys and one girl to church very faithfully almost every Sunday. They were well-behaved children, pleasant, quiet, with slow smiles, always dressed neatly. As the boys got old enough, they served as acolytes and occasionally, with their mother, as ushers.

We made arrangements for Blair to be treated by Dr. Books once or twice a month, as their family budget would allow. He came to my home with his head hung low and tilted to one side, his shoulders curled forward. He didn't want to look me in the face. He stuttered and couldn't pronounce some of the letters. It was not because he didn't try or that his parents had not tried to help him. And it was not that the school speech therapist had not tried. His tongue just could not move correctly to get the words out.

How did Dr. Books treat Blair? She worked just a little on his posture and on balancing his body framework because his body balance was pretty good; rather, in his case, she worked primarily with his tongue. She actually took hold of his tongue and moved it around in his mouth. Using a very gentle pressure she worked on his jaws to make room in his mouth for his tongue to move freely and to rest properly behind the teeth. Therefore, with only a few gentle treatments she was able to adjust his face, head, and jaws.

After six half-hour treatments over seven months—NO MORE STUTTER-ING! Blair pronounced the words clearly! He no longer hung his head in shame. It seemed like a miracle to me. During that time Blair celebrated his ninth birthday.

Four years later, on a Sunday morning, I spoke with Blair—who had grown taller than I—and another young teenager. He joined in the conversation freely and spoke clearly. Instead of going off to the playground to play alone, he now joins in the activities of the youth group. The amazing thing was that he did not remember how he used to stutter. He is doing so well that the problems of the past have been forgotten. Now he is thinking about what he wants to be when he finishes school.

Did you ever stop to think what a wonderful gift from God the ability to forget is? How terrible life would be if we remembered all the aches and pains we suffered during our lifetimes. What a blessing that Blair could forget that he used to stutter when he was younger.

Talking with Blair's mother I learned that he no longer was in speech therapy classes. That is a big savings to the school district. Wouldn't it be wonderful if all the children who stutter could be helped by Books Neural Therapy™ so that with only a little speech therapy they could speak clearly and without embarrassment? It could save the school districts money, the families a lot of worries, and the children much frustration.

11

Do you know a family where several generations have TROUBLE READING? This family did.

This family—mother, father, and daughter—came in for a treatment. There were two daughters in the family. The younger one was very well-adjusted, the older, Melissa, now a teenager was frustrated because she could not perform according to her family's expectations. Her parents were professional, well educated, charming, and held prominent places in their community.

The father came along because he wanted to experience the results of a treatment. He discovered he felt so much better after one treatment. The mother, a talented lady, was very good at relating to people one-on-one, but had a difficult time in large groups. She expressed a desire to be more at ease in front of large gatherings. When she was young she suffered a severe fall on her tailbone; this kind of fall often causes problems with learning, such as **dyslexia.** This seemed to be the result in this mother. Handwriting was difficult for her; she tended to reverse letters and words. **Dyslexics** often reverse letters in words such as "saw" instead of "was". This can cause embarrassment in front of a class, but can be cleverly covered up most of the time. Her class work, when she was still in school, was inconsistent—one day she would know the lesson, the next day, the same lesson, she would not. After her treatments with Dr. Books she felt much better and was able to perform better.

Melissa, the daughter, felt like she was on the outside, as if she did not fit in. She could not reach the standards set by her younger sister. She neglected her personal appearance because she did not see herself as attractive. She kept her head down and would not look us in the eye. Junior high school was a struggle, and because she had problems with schoolwork, she was put in special classes. During the summer she attended a camp where she had power reading courses.

Melissa loved horseback riding, backpacking, power walking, and skiing. She was very good, one-on-one, with people.

Her parents reported that before meeting Dr. Books, Melissa was very **depressed**. After her treatments were completed I received a lovely note from her parents. It said, "Dear Bernice, Thank you so much for bringing Dr. Books to us. She has opened doors to us all, and I am very grateful to her and to you for this gift. You are a special lady. Sincerely, James and Family". The family saw many positive improvements in their daughter, both in her schoolwork and her relationships with other people.

After graduating from high school, Melissa moved to New York to attend college. During her college years, Melissa visited Bombay and Bangalore, India, where she made two documentary films on the subject, "Women's Health Care as It Exists in India". She graduated from Brooklyn College with a degree in Film and Video.

Now she is employed at a digital processing company in New York, and is doing very well.

12

Do you know people who are ACCIDENT PRONE? CHRISTIAN AND HIS MOTHER WERE

The townspeople in our Danish tourist village were assembling for the annual Danish Sisterhood Christmas party. Garlands and Danish Christmas hearts hung on the walls of the parish hall and an eighteen-foot Monterey pine Christmas tree, decorated with lights and balls, stood in the center. Tables were covered with red tablecloths; white napkins enclosed the knife, fork, and spoon. Centerpieces were Christmas evergreens interspersed with votive candles sparkling inside little glass globes.

A young man sat at a table across the room from me. He had long, straight hair reaching below his collar, and very delicate features. He looked familiar. Pretty soon he saw me and got up and walked over to my table. It was Christian. Although I had known him since he was a young boy, I had not seen him for almost two years. Five years earlier Christian, a student at UCSB, was having a difficult time getting through college because of his **learning disabilities**. He came to see Dr. Books, complaining of **headaches**, and **reading difficulties**.

Like so many people with learning difficulties Christian had walked, a little stooped over, in a strange gait—almost like a duck's waddle. One shoulder was lower than the other, and his right ear was higher on his head than his left ear. He told how he had been knocked unconscious in a skateboard accident when he was younger. He also had difficulties with **allergies**, was clumsy and **accident prone**, had poor self-esteem, and found it difficult to complete projects. He expressed a problem with handwriting, memory, and with vision—which was eventually corrected by laser surgery. Conditions such as these are often caused by neurological problems, in Christian's case it was in his mandible joint causing **temporoman-**

dibular joint pain dysfunction syndrome (TMJ). Dr. Books was able to correct his problems with only six "Books Neural Therapy™" treatments.

I was thrilled to see the young man who stood before me now. He was tall—over six feet—and stood erect. His body was balanced, and his shoulders were even. He spoke clearly, with confidence; his thoughts were well organized. His charming wife and cute little daughter came over with him to meet me. He spoke proudly of his family and his job in the computer industry in Santa Barbara. The changes in Christian's life seemed like a miracle to Christian, his family, and to me.

When Christian came to see Dr. Books he was accompanied by his mother, Velma. At the time she was straining to finish college; she tended to skip over her work and could not remember what she had learned. Like her son she was **accident-prone** and had **allergies**. She had trouble reading her own handwriting, writing that wandered on the page. She also struggled with self-esteem.

Her difficulties seemed to result from a whiplash in an auto accident. As a child she fell a lot, and continued to do so as an adult, because she had poor depth perception. She often bumped her head. As a result she suffered from a lot of **depression**.

Velma had many "Books Neural Therapy™" treatments from Dr. Books. After that it was like she had a complete new body. She was very lovely, self-assured, and confident. It seemed like a miracle to both Velma and to me.

The treatments will last a lifetime if there is no further trauma, such as a bad fall or an auto accident that could knock or throw the body off balance again. Dr. Books likes people to come in for "tune ups" first on a monthly basis, then quarterly, then yearly. Even with all her degrees and credentials, she keeps learning new things about the brain, the body and learning. She is eager to keep everyone as fit as possible and learning as easily as possible

13

Have you ever noticed that among siblings there are many similairities, while at the same time there are definite differences? Here is one such sibling, BRAD.

When God makes people he makes all different kinds. Some are tall. Some are short. Some are thin. Some are fat. Some are doctors or lawyers. Some are farmers or auto mechanics. Some are artists. Some are musicians. Some are firemen. Some are policemen. We need different kinds of people with different talents and different abilities to make our communities function.

That is what makes this world such an interesting place. However, when these people are little children, they don't all fit in the same mold as they go through school. Even in the same family, children have different interests and different personalities.

Brad was 10 years old and in the fifth grade when he entered our summer 2001 program. His sister Marcia was 8 years old and in grade three.

Brad had a positive attitude. He was cheerful, considerate, bright and thoughtful. Encouragement was needed to get his homework in on time, stay focused on a task and work independently. Those around him treated him with kindness, patience and support.

Brad enjoys music and martial arts. In writing, his letters were poorly formed. Poor eye hand coordination made sports difficult for him. Math was challenging for him. Learning the multiplication tables was arduous. He said that "His eyes go blank at times."

Among Brad's problems were following multiple instructions given at one time, confusing right and left, sometimes reversing numbers and letters. Concentrating was extremely difficult unless it was something he was very interested in.

At age seven Brad had endured three seizures. He was tested with an EEG and MRI. The MRI was negative. Sensory Perception Examination showed mild imbalance, struggle with standing or hopping on either foot; poor heal to toe walking, and difficulty interposing fingers. Also during the course of childhood Brad suffered from pneumonia, allergies and mild asthma. For relief from the allergies he was treated by Dr. Sobyl Bunis D.C. (Who also uses the NAET allergy elimination technique that Dr. Books uses.) As a toddler of only 13 months Brad had tubes in his ears for ear infections.

Brad's goals for his summer treatments with Dr. Phyllis Books were to be able to concentrate better, without any medication, and to not feel overloaded with information. Brad wanted to improve in math and make his homework easier, not to be so stressed, and not get distracted when trying to do his schoolwork.

Brad enjoyed 18 treatments from Dr. Books during July and August of 2001.

In the Wide Range Achievement Test (WRAT) conducted before and after treatments Brad improved one grade level in arithmetic, reading and spelling. In the Bruininks-Oseretsky test of gross and fine motor skills Brad improved from the 38th percentile to the 90th percentile. In the Test Of Variables of Attention (T.O.V.A.) Brad improved his ADHD score from -4.76 to -3.06 a 35.7% improvement. (Normal range is -1.00 to +1.00).

For three years from 2001 to 2004 Brad's mom and dad home schooled their children. Now they are in regular school again.

Brad saw and felt the positive results of Dr. Books work on him self. He learned to organize himself. His grades improved. He is doing well in his regular high school classes but is struggling with his honors classes.

Electronics, inventions, video games, and reading are some of the things that Brad now enjoys. Sociability, kindness and gentleness are some of his fine qualities. His parents are good role models and supportive.

His ambition is to go to a four year college and become a writer. Brad taught himself some tools to cope with his ADD and only takes medication if he is facing a problem that requires special focus. If he is having problems with his Allergies again, he will ask to go to Dr. Bunis. Her practice is in Santa Barbara, Santa Ynez and San Luis Obispo.

14

Have you ever noticed that among siblings there are many similarities, while at the same time there are definite differences? Here is a second sibling, Marcia.

Chapter 13 is about Marcia's brother Brad. In Chapter 14 we will take a look at his younger sister, Marcia.

Marcia was 8 years old and in grade 3 when she joined our summer 2001 California program.

Marcia is personable, sociable, outgoing, and athletic. She likes basketball, soccer, gymnastics and tennis. Ballet and jazz dance classes also provide enjoyment. Her private art lessons are a treat for her. She is a bright and active learner when she likes the subject and the teacher.

The problem is, she has difficulty paying attention and staying focused on her work. She used to use her fingers to help her with her math. It was hard for her to hold sequential thoughts. Listening and following instructions was a dilemma for her, especially in math.

In first and second grade if she got hurt physically, or was frustrated, she would want to go home. Sometimes she displayed a quick temper. When she was in a bad mood it was difficult to get anything done.

From those around her Marcia is treated with kindness and support. Her parents are good role models. But if she gets upset and doesn't know how to do some things she just shuts down. Her compulsive behavior almost causes her to get hurt.

Marcia may cooperate with one teacher, but not with another. If she likes a subject she will stay focused, if not, she will day dream. Marcia was diagnosed with ADHD and takes Ritalin.

Marcia's goals with Dr. Books' treatments were to be able to concentrate better without medication, to be able to follow simple instructions, like brush your teeth, get dressed, and to improve her reading.

On her Bruininks-Oseretsky pre and post test, which is gross and fine motor skills (and I like to make a game of it), which were done before and after her 18 treatments with Dr. Books, Marcia improved from the 62nd percentile to the 97th percentile. Great job!

On her T.O.V.A. Test of variables of attention she improved from minus - 2.54 to plus +1.58. This shows how good she can be when she wants to be.

I could never understand why her scores went down on her Wide Range Achievement Test until her mother told me about her shutting down if she doesn't like something. I found a short note on the back of her test from the teacher who gave the test to her saying she had decided to shut down and refused to complete the WRAT portion of the post-test.

There is such a difference in children.

15

ADD, ALLERGIES, DYSLEXIA, DEVELOPMENTALY DELAYED,
You have problems?
MARTIN did.

Martin spent his school year with his father in Wisconsin; in the summer he came to California to stay with his mother. Martin was awkward, jerky in his movements and walked with an unbalanced gait because the neurological pathways from his brain to his muscles were not coordinated. One early diagnosis of his condition was: "Learning disabled and developmentally delayed".

He learned to ride a two-wheeler at six years of age, so his balance was good then. Subsequent falls on his head and on his tailbone knocked him out of alignment and contributed to some of his problems. At age eight Martin had an EEG and an EKG, which indicated conductive problems. Also at eight he had eye muscle surgery. When he was nine he had a bicycle accident and had to have stitches close a cut over his eye. At ten he had a heart murmur and was diagnosed with Attention Deficit Disorder (ADD) and hyperactivity. At eleven he had a second bike accident and bruised his nose and eye. Another indication of lack of muscle control was that he was not able to control his bowels. Either he was constipated or would lose control.

Sports were good physical exercise and fun, but he was clumsy, accident-prone, had balance problems and poor motor coordination—and the fact that he had difficulty following instructions meant that he wasn't very good at sports.

When he was fifteen he was still reading at the second grade level. Vision problems and dyslexia made reading, spelling, writing, and arithmetic difficult. He had problems concentrating and remembering to do such things as turning in his homework and completing projects. He had a hard time saying what he meant, especially when asked questions, which made his self-esteem very low. To help he would ask people to repeat what they said. Martin was allergic to dairy products, corn, wheat, sugar, and substitute sweeteners.

As he got older his frustrations increased because he wanted to be out with other children, yet he could not react as they did. He enjoyed drawing, wood-working, playing video games, bike riding, and playing with Legos.

After a summer of treatments with Dr. Books both of his eyes moved together, which made it possible for him to maintain eye contact with other people instead of looking at the ground. This increased his self-confidence and encouraged more verbal interaction. Dr. Books treated him for his allergies, which made his life more pleasant. The painless method Dr. Books uses for eliminating allergies is called NAET: Nambudripad's Allergy Elimination Technique. Dr. Nambudri-pad, who developed this wonderful procedure, came to the United States from India.

When Martin went back to Wisconsin to school in the fall he looked better, which helped his self-esteem. He walked erect, with smooth movements. He appeared more balanced. His schoolwork improved, much to the delight of his teachers. His mother received an email from his teacher telling how much he had improved over the summer. Instead of figuring out ways to avoid his schoolwork he sat right down and did it immediately. The improvements in Martin seemed like a miracle to his mother, his teachers and to me.

Martin's mother was so impressed with the improvements in her son during the brief time he was in California that, after an accident that resulted in pains in her head and spine, she came to Dr. Books for treatments. Her body was gently moved back into correct position so that she was no longer in pain.

Martin is one of the examples of children who keep improving over time. Like some other patients, Martin continued to see Dr. Books whenever they were both in Solvang at the same time. His developmental delays eventually were overcome.

Martin graduated from high school with honors because he exceeded all his IEP goals. He won several awards for racing quads in Wisconsin. After high school Martin started working with his father in construction.

16

Has someone you know thought about attempting SUICIDE? Dennis did.

o o o o o o o o o o o o o o o o o o o o o o o o o o o o o o o o

"I tried to commit suicide five times. I tried slashing my wrists and taking ant poison."

Dr. Books called me one day from Dallas to tell me about a patient in Oakland, California, who needed help. She had such confidence in me, and my hospitality, that she made arrangements for this young man to come to Solvang for treatments without first asking me. Of course I said, "Okay."

Even though he was twenty-one years old, the patient, Dennis, did not drive (he could read very little so he could not get a driver's license); therefore, it would be too difficult for him to get around in Dallas. Solvang is much smaller and much closer to Dennis's home in Northern California.

Dennis's father lived in San Diego. Dr. Books told his father that Dennis could stay at my house and she would treat him here—two treatments in the morning, one in the afternoon—and I would tutor him in between. Of course the father was a little leery about who I might be, so he called me to get acquainted and asked the best way for Dennis to get to Solvang. I suggested that Dennis take the Amtrak Bus, which would bring him directly from Oakland to Solvang, where I would pick him up.

I asked his father how I would recognize his son, and he described him as being tall, well built, muscular, with a mustache, a little beard, with a short haircut similar to a buzz. He also wears gold-rimmed glasses, and is black. I responded, "Okay, I'll look for a tall, handsome young man with a good suntan".

Dennis's father laughed and felt more at ease about letting his son come to my home. Dennis, of course, was a little hesitant, but he trusted that his dad knew what was best for him. Dennis's mother had come from Ghana, Africa, where his father and mother met at the university. His father is an engineer. His mother is an accountant.

It was very dark that Saturday night about ten o'clock when Dennis got off the bus. I brought him home and made him comfortable in his room. Then I asked him to fill in the application form that Dr. Books asks of all her clients. He was able to fill in only a few of the blanks.

Sunday morning he cheerfully went to church with us. Dennis told me that he enjoyed going to church with one of his friends and his friend's parents in Northern California. Since his parents were divorced, Dennis had little sense of family. During the previous ten years of his life, conversations with his father had never been very deep.

Dennis was a very God-centered, faithful Christian. In youth activities, such as Young Life, he learned to love God as his Heavenly Father. Trips to Mexico with Young Life, to help build homes for the poor, were the kinds of activities he really enjoyed. He told me about helping to build a small house for a mother, father, and three children who had been living in three panels of wood nailed together. The new three-room house with a cement floor, roof, and four walls seemed like a palace for the Mexican family. This experience gave Dennis a lot of self-esteem and helped him to appreciate what he had in his life, despite his parents' divorce. His parents always provided good clothes to wear, good food to eat, and a nice place to live.

That Sunday afternoon I helped him fill in the rest of the form. After that I had him read to me so that I could see what his reading level was; and I had him do some math. He read very slowly with much difficulty. I had him read a Dr. Seuss book, which is usually easy for children, but he struggled with many of the words. Then I had him try to read the *Reader's Digest*; he would get frustrated and skip the difficult words. Since he was familiar with religious vocabulary I had him read a religious magazine; he did a little better with that. I checked his math ability. He did all right with simple addition, but when I asked him to subtract eighty from a hundred he had a very difficult time doing it.

Dennis told how he had Attention Deficit Disorder (ADD) and was in special education all through school. He was teased and called bad names by other children. He had been treated by a regular chiropractor off and on for three years, but the treatments hurt; he did not like them and they were not helping. As a result he was very leery of trying a new treatment that involved a chiropractor. Nevertheless, his dad convinced him he should try, so here he was.

Dennis was determined that his learning disability was not going to keep him out of everything he wanted to do. In order to learn by doing, he took all the after-school activities and programs available. He visited convalescent homes and helped with younger children after school and at summer camps. Even though he could not do the schoolwork himself he encouraged the children to do their work just by his presence, smile, and kind words. Dennis developed memory skills that allowed him to memorize a lot of Scripture. He had also memorized a speech that Mark Twain gave one Fourth of July in England. Dennis was invited to recite this speech at summer camps and various meetings, using the Mark Twain dialect, and was very clever at doing it.

When Dennis told us about his problems in reading, eye-hand coordination, math, writing (he was still printing and not writing cursive), his frustration was evident. Before Dr. Books started treating him on Sunday afternoon, Dennis was five-feet-ten-and-one-eighth inches tall. When we had him walk down the hall, his gait was not as bad as some people's, but we could see that his right hip was lower than his left, his shoulders were not balanced, his hands hung at different lengths, and he had that slight tilt to his walk that many learning disabled people have. He read at about a third-grade level, doing pretty well on one-syllable words. But when he came to longer words that he couldn't figure out he would get disgusted and skip them.

He knew how to add and subtract, but did not know how to multiply or divide. When I asked him to multiply 3x7 he answered, "23". Asked to add 7+7, his first answer was "18," then he tried it on his fingers and got 14. So I said, "Add 7 more" he came up with 20. We finally got to 3x7=21. When I told him to take 80 from 100, he asked, "Is that minus?" It took him quite a while to figure out the answer.

Putting large numbers into words was impossible. Words like four, ten, or seven, he was able to spell, but he could not spell amounts in dollars, or numbers in the thousands or millions. He did not know how to write the symbol for division. We continued to do a little exploring until I could see where he was academically.

I asked, "What is your favorite Bible passage?" While he was thinking, I started John 3:16, "For God so...," he quickly quoted the rest of it. He told the story of the rich young ruler in Luke 18 in his own words quite well.

After I tested Dennis, Dr. Books began her work on him, feeling his neck and shoulders and seeing where his imbalances were. She started on the foundation of the body, his feet. Dennis had unusual feet. He did not have arches as most people do, the arch actually extended outward rather than inward and Dennis's toe muscles were very stiff.

(Remember the rhyme you recite when you play with a child's toes as you wiggle them back and forth?

> This little piggy went to market, this little piggy stayed home,
> This little piggy had roast beef, this little piggy had none,
> This little piggy cried 'wee, wee, wee' all the way home.

This is an important nursery rhyme to play with your little ones. Wiggling those little toes on babies and little children helps stimulate the brain activity. Don't ask me how it works, all I know is that it does. It is important that the toes be able to wiggle and move. That is why it is important that children's shoes allow them to grow. When you buy shoes for your children you should allow a thumb's width at the front of the shoe to allow for growth. Cramping the toes in shoes that are too small can cause misshapen feet, and other problems.)

Dr. Books continued from Dennis's toes to his ankles and Achilles tendons, to his legs, hips, and pelvis. The hips and pelvic area are the framework of the body. You cannot put a roof on a house until the foundation and framework are finished; structure and function go together.

As Dr. Books' hands moved gently up the spine she found that Dennis had very slight scoliosis (lateral curvature of the spine). Then she moved on to the scapula (the shoulder blades) and to the tender spots on his neck. When she got to Dennis's skull she held it very patiently as if she were holding a chord on the piano, pressing her fingers on various spots where the bones meet. She manipulated his ears to improve coordination between the eyes and the ears. As is often the case, the temporomandibular joint also needed adjusting; with sterile protectors on her fingers she worked on the lower jaw inside his mouth. When all else was in balance, she massaged around the eye muscles.

Dennis could not move his eyes up and down without moving his full forehead and lower jaw. He tried his best but he had to use his forehead and jaw to move his eyes. Dr. Books very gently released the tension in the muscles around his eyes so that he could move them up and down and back and forth without the help from his forehead and jaw.

Each day, for the next five days, Dr. Books treated Dennis in a half-hour session twice each morning and once each afternoon, going over the same routine, so that eventually the muscles and bones of Dennis's body would respond and stay where they belonged. I tutored him in between with reading—especially with the alphabet—handwriting, and mathematics.

After fifteen treatments over a period of five days, Dennis was half an inch taller than he was when he began the treatments; his walk was more even, his shoulders more level, and his hands hung evenly at his side. His reading had improved about three grade levels. Now he read with expression, joy, and ease, comprehending at about the sixth-grade level rather than the third. When he came to a word he was not sure of he could figure it out by himself, which made him feel very happy. Now he could read just for the joy of reading, whereas before he hated to read, because the symbols just didn't make sense to him.

His dad had said that his own goal was to receive a short note, written by Dennis, that he could read and understand. After his treatments Dennis wrote, in large print, a letter to his dad. It was not perfect, but it was more than he had ever been able to do before.

1-26-00

Dear Dad,

I am doing well here in Solvang. Things seem to be working out here with the treatment with Dr. Books. So I thing it is all work out here of Solvang at Bernice house but I think it has to due with prayer it has alot to due with if I due say so myself becues when we put God first in our lifes all things are possible with God but with out God nothing seem to work so the power of God's hand is at work here. I can feel it in every place in Solvang and mosetliy in me and Dad I can see it all over Bernice and in Dr. books. The love of God. Here are some of the things that have changed in my life. Before I so hated to read things in books but now I love to read I cant even put book down till reading more then 20 pg or sometime even more than that. It may be hard for you to believe that but it is true. Thanks to God and Dr. Books and Bernice. I can write better and clearer. I am better at my math now. Dr. Books asked me to write a naote a small note to you and I cant stop writeing this letter to you Dad. Thanks alot for making this possible. You son alwas good bye.

P.S. cant wait to see you and Delores in a couple of weeks. Dennis.

He could barely read before he came to Solvang. But after fifteen treatments of Books Neural Therapy™ he could read thirty pages at a sitting, and his math and writing had improved as well. He was so excited about his new abilities; he felt it was like a miracle. He said, "People who don't know God, don't know how many miracles can happen."

Dennis is a very polite young man, very well mannered. He showed his appreciation by being thoughtful and faithful in following instructions.

Four months after his treatments, Dr. Books and I met with Dennis and his father in San Diego. We interviewed Dennis and his father to see how Books Neural Therapy™ had changed his life. He then opened up to us about some of the sad things that had happened in his life and how difficult and unhappy his childhood had been because he could not succeed in school the way he wanted to. He knew he was not dumb, it was just that he could not see things the way other people did. He had a good mind, he could memorize, he had a good voice and could speak, but he could not do math or spell or read and was frustrated in school because those are the things we are expected to accomplish in school. He was so miserable, in fact, that he had tried to commit **suicide** five times.

Suicide is alarmingly common. Dr. Books has ways of assessing self-destructive patterns in certain misalignments of the cranial and sacral (head and tailbone) areas. Patients freely discuss their attempted suicides and suicidal thoughts with Dr. Books, grateful that someone is noticing their distress. (For most patients this is very confidential. Dennis talked about it openly.) Before Dr. Books' treatments Dennis felt as if he were in a box with a bunch of tigers and couldn't get out.

I interviewed Dennis's father who admitted to having some of the same problems when he was a child. It was painful for him to talk about it because it brought back so many memories. He admitted not spending a lot of time with his son because it was hard to face his son having the same problems he had endured. In a way, he had sacrificed his father-son relationship to avoid his own pain. However, once his son wrote that letter to him his heart started melting. He said, "I feel like I've got my son back."

Two years later I phoned Dennis to see how he was doing. He was working as a teaching assistant at a new high school. The students he worked with had problems such as blindness, or other long-term disabilities. He helped the children get around the campus and get their assignments from their teachers. The children are smart but have physical problems that require assistance; they are in regular classes most of the day and have one "special" period. Dennis felt this was much better for the students than being in Special Ed classes all day. He is very encouraging, a good role model, and the children like him. Being a yard supervisor at the school is fun for him.

Recently, Dennis returned from a trip to Baja Mexico, his fifth time with Young Life, along with a group of three hundred Christian young people. They volunteered for a week in Mexico to build ten houses. The Mexican families who had been living in cardboard shelters with dirt floors now had houses with concrete slab floors, poured before the Young Life group arrived. The young people helped put up the framing, plywood exterior walls, dry-wall interior walls, with tarpaper and shingle roofs, for the ten three-room-and-loft homes. They installed wiring for electricity even though there is no electricity in the area yet. They also dug a ten-foot-deep latrine for each family, a change from the one latrine for the whole community. There is no running water available in the area.

Helping build these homes was a very rewarding experience for Dennis because he could do something positive for others. He feels very good about that and it also makes him appreciate his own home, with electricity, running water, and indoor plumbing.

In February 2002, Dennis went to Australia for a month to visit a friend he had met in San Diego two years before. To earn spending money while in Australia, Dennis picked cotton and discovered what hard work is. During the previous summer Dennis worked at "Wolf Burro," a Boy Scout camp in the mountains near Lake Tahoe. He helped with cooking, served as chaplain, as ranger, and was so well liked that they asked him to stay on longer.

Dennis sounded very happy with his life at that point. Things were going well for him.

17

Do you have problems with DYSLEXIA, PERCEPTION, or MISUNDERSTANDING? MARJORIE did.

Marjorie, a petite, attractive fifty-seven-year-old told us that she was **dyslexic** and had problems with **perception** and **understanding**. Marjorie had seen Dr. Books years earlier; but now she drove five hours and spent a week in Solvang, so that Dr. Books could address deeper issues that were surfacing during some advanced life coaching training. A slight hearing loss had been treated with acupuncture. Her list of past physical problems included: pneumonia, allergies, broken bones, problems during menopause, and now she experienced joint pain, neck pain, back pain between her shoulders, muscle stiffness, muscle cramps, and other problems with her feet, ankles, and hips. Despite all of these she enjoyed swimming, kayaking, walking, and dancing.

Describing herself as an introvert she said she worked around it to study whatever would contribute to her personal growth. Marjorie is very good at intuitive counseling, but finds group presentations difficult.

When she was a child in school she found that math was hard for her; she did not have a good memory and had trouble concentrating and following instructions, especially if she received multiple instructions all at once, and often had to have people repeat what they said. She would sometimes get lost because she confused left and right directions. Her family had her tested to see why she was having these problems. In those days, when not much was known about learning disabilities, they could not reach any conclusions. Marjorie, in an effort to compensate, took a lot of extra reading courses.

She came to Dr. Books for two series of "Books Neural Therapy™" treatments to see if they could correct her **dyslexic** tendencies, show her how to process information, and help her overcome her deep fear base. After the second treatment she felt "comfortable" inside her body, just as she wanted to feel. It is hard for other people to understand this feeling; sometimes it is like being a prisoner inside your own body. You want to escape but you can't. Dr. Books gently adjusted her body so her neurological system could connect properly. When this is done, pain is eased and the body can begin to function optimally.

This procedure is not common to all chiropractors because it is beyond what is taught in chiropractic schools. Additional studies in nutrition, psychology, as well as certain European and Asian disciplines are needed. Some problems are common to most people and can be treated the same. But every situation involves a combination of treatment types. And each treatment has to be tailored to each individual patient, depending on each person's body and its problems.

Marjorie felt as if she had received a miracle after all those years of suffering.

As a postscript to Marjorie's experience, she felt a special connection to Dr. Books after watching her treat Tim, her twenty-six-year-old mentally retarded son. As with Marjorie's decision to seek care for her self, there was an earlier time when it seemed appropriate for her to seek care for Tim.

Tim was working at a fast-food restaurant at the time and doing pretty well. However, Marjorie sensed, after working with Dr. Books herself, that Dr. Books had something to offer her son. Like many patients, Dr. Books did an initial series of treatments and would do tune-ups whenever she was in town for Tim.

One day, while working on eye-tracking issues, she saw a funny look pass over his face; out of nowhere she found herself asking him, "Do you feel responsible for your parent's divorce?" Although he had been sitting, he flopped down on the treatment table, as if an arrow pierced through his heart. He seemed relieved and distraught at the same time.

Dr. Books immediately changed gears and went through some forgiveness exercises while she gently continued to hold him and work with him. He repeated the forgiveness phrases to himself over and over until he fell asleep with forgiveness on his lips. His mother was weeping in the corner. She offered to pay double for the session, saying no amount of money could ever pay for the miracle she just witnessed.

18

Do you know someone who was at a DETENTION Facility and went on to COLLEGE? MIKE did.

I met Mike through a friend of mine who was concerned about him because he had made some foolish mistakes and got himself in trouble. When Mike was in junior high school he got into fights, was rebellious, and eventually was kicked out of junior high. Opportunity schools were his next option; when that didn't work he was sent to Los Prietos Boys Camp (a detention facility in the mountains for teenage boys in minor trouble with the law) where attempts are made to straighten out young offenders. Their treatment includes one-half day of physical work and one-half day of schoolwork, but this does not straighten out their bodies, their minds, or their spirits.

The primary problem is that these boys need to be straightened out physically, neurologically, mentally, and emotionally, before they can expect to be law-abiding citizens. That is why so many young men who start out in the juvenile court system end up in the adult court system. They need to have their bodies actually straightened out and balanced, so they can function properly. Some people reflect this problem by the way they walk; they are crooked, out of balance, and slouch from side to side as well as forward. Statistics range from: 60–90 percent of adult prisoners are functionally illiterate; and 95 percent of boys in juvenile detention facilities have trouble reading.

When Mike walked his hips clicked, his legs popped and he had very flat feet. As a result he'd had a number of falls and accidents. He had vision problems and his jaw clicked. As a child he had asthma and allergies. Leukemia at the age of eight required him to have bone-marrow transplants and spinal taps. After four years he recovered and showed no signs of it now. He also endured a lot of back pain.

Emotional and mental stress also complicated Mike's life. The relationship with his own father was minimal; his father and brother were addicted to heroin and marijuana so Mike tried to stay away from his own home and live with my friend as much as possible, sharing a father-son relationship with my friend's husband. This family often included him in their activities, which gave him a feeling of connectedness.

Thanks to the Assisi scholarship fund Mike was actually able to get fourteen treatments from Dr. Books. He was very grateful for this opportunity and thankful that someone cared about him and paid attention to him. His goal was to improve the movement of his body with less pain and stress. When he completed his treatments, at the age of twenty, he was without pain, and had his head on straight. His reading skills improved from freshman level to senior level in high school. In spelling he improved from fifth to tenth grade level, and in arithmetic he improved from eighth grade to tenth grade.

The following summer he got a job in construction. In the fall he enrolled at Santa Barbara City College. This relief from pain and scholastic improvement seemed like a miracle to Mike and to his friends.

One of our original goals in the Assisi scholarship program was to actually go into Los Prietos Boys Camp and treat twenty of the boys who were detained there. We wanted to show how these treatments could reduce the crime rate and save the taxpayers money. By releasing these boys from the prison of their own bodies—physically, structurally, neurologically, and emotionally—they could become productive members of society, rather than continuing on to a life of crime. Unfortunately, by the time we raised the money, the staff person in control at the Sheriff's Department with whom we'd made arrangements had moved on; his replacement did not allow us in. How sad for the boys and for society.

Statistics vary around the country, indicating that anywhere from 60% to 90% of the people in jail can not read well enough to hold a good job. Wouldn't it be great if we could cut those numbers in half by using Books Neural Therapy™ to adjust their bodies so they could be successful?

* Mike is number 9 in the California Research Project 2001 Spring Group

19

Do you know someone who is plagued with MENTAL, EMOTIONAL, AND PHYSICAL STRESS? JOE was.

Joe was fourteen when he came to my house for treatments, and in the ninth grade. He also had spent time at Los Prietos Camp for boys (as mentioned in earlier chapters, Los Prietos is a correctional facility in the nearby mountains for teenage boys.)

Joe had a slight build and an almost defiant manner, contrary to the kind of downtrodden expression many learning-disabled people have. Joe's family had a history of ADD, addiction, and depression. When his mother was pregnant with him she was under a lot of physical, emotional, and financial stress, so she smoked. His brother suffered from depression, and Joe, due to the loss of loved ones and changes in his life situation, was suffering mental and emotional stress.

Periodically Joe would become **disoriented** and get lost. Sometimes he felt **dizzy** and would lose his balance. He was **accident-prone** and he'd had several bad falls. After his second bicycle accident in four years he was taken to the hospital with a head injury (requiring four staples in his head) and temporary amnesia. To compound his problems, he also had a degenerating disease of his spine causing both lower and upper back pain. He also had pain in his knees.

Joe's learning disability showed up in his reading and concentration. It was difficult for him to follow instructions, especially if he was given two or three orders at a time. He would often ask teachers to repeat what they had just said. Most kids, if asked a question, would give some kind of answer, believing they had a fifty-fifty chance of being right. Joe would be hesitant to guess and would just not answer. Consequently he became rebellious and would act up or make trouble to divert attention from the fact that he did not know what he was supposed to do.

Joe often reversed numbers or letters, a symptom of **dyslexia**. He would forget to finish his homework or forget to turn it in if he did finish it. When he tried to talk, occasionally the words he meant to say would not come out, so he could not always express himself. According to some analysts, Joe "showed a deficit in his ability to synthesize concrete parts into meaningful wholes." In other words, he could not put syllables together to make whole words. Joe was in special education classes from the fourth to eighth grades. He did not take his high school proficiency test and was given remedial work.

Joe's mother had been to Dr. Books for treatments, so she knew how helpful the treatments could be and how much better she felt. Joe had a rather haphazard attitude toward the work that Dr. Books and I were trying to do with him. So I took him into a room by himself and explained that I was working very hard raising money so that he could be helped free of charge, and I was very disappointed that he did not want to take advantage of this gift. People had donated lots of money so that he and others could have this opportunity. If he did not want to take advantage of this, then I would find someone else who did. After that he shaped up and started to cooperate with the doctor and me.

Joe's first "Wide Range Achievement Test", taken in March before any treatments, showed that he read at a fourth-grade level. After sixteen one-half hour treatments of "Books Neural Therapy™", his reading test score improved to a twelfth-grade level. In arithmetic he had scored at seventh-grade level, now, after treatments, at eleventh-grade level. He did not do as well in spelling. However, his mother was very, very happy to see the academic, physical, and social improvements in Joe. The results of Dr. Books work on this young man seemed like a miracle to me and to his mother. His mother's therapist called Dr. Books and set up a luncheon to discuss what in the world she was doing that no one else had been able to do.

* Joe is number 6 in the California Research Project 2001 Spring Group.

20

Do you have friends who have a MYSTERIOUS PAIN, COPPER TOXICITY or DYSLEXIA? TORONTO & TRACEY did.

Who is this tall, nice looking man, dressed in cowboy boots, jeans, western shirt, and Stetson hat ringing my doorbell? Looks like a motion picture cowboy. It was Toronto, a bona fide movie cowboy whose favorite pastime is horseback riding. In his career he had been bounced around so much, and had so many falls and other accidents, both in his work in the movies and while riding for pleasure, that he was now in a **lot of pain**.

Although he had originally seen Dr. Books for treatments in Texas, now he had come to my house to see if Dr. Books could relieve the misery in his head, neck, and body. When his treatments started, sometimes he would drive to Solvang early in the morning, get a treatment, then drive back to Los Angeles to work by noon. Toronto's girlfriend, Tracey, would sometimes come with him for treatments. She was suffering from whiplash pains as the result of an auto accident. This petite, charming actress worked in the movies when assignments were available, but her steady job was as a College teacher.

As a clinical nutritionist, Dr. Books will take a hair sample from certain patients who are difficult to diagnose and send it out to be tested. The lab will test for fifty different minerals. Dr. Books took a sample of Tracey's hair and sent it to an analytical research lab in Phoenix, Arizona, to see if she had a **chemical imbalance**. The tests showed that she had a number of mineral imbalances, including an excess of copper to the extent that she had **copper toxicity**, which affects the thyroid and adrenal glands and often induces mood problems.

People with this disorder are often prone to disorders such as **dyslexia**. Copper has a stimulatory effect upon the neuro transmitters that control many brain functions. Tracey was also deficient in zinc, and her calcium-magnesium ratio was out of order so that she was not able to metabolize sugars and simple carbohydrates, allowing her to eat big meals, yet remain very slim. According to the lab, her high calcium level served as a protective device, a calcium shell to block off physical and emotional stress caused by copper toxicity. She was not getting enough meat protein, so the lab suggested that she increase her meat protein intake to improve the effect of her thyroid and adrenal glands.

Research shows that an excess of sugar and refined foods may deplete chromium reserves. She had a low chromium reserve which is an essential trace mineral involved in fat protein and carbohydrate metabolism regulation, so she needed to add organ meat and brewers yeast to her diet.

Blood tests are good for testing many problems, but heavy metals are best reviewed by hair analysis. The lab in Phoenix provides a very detailed but easy to understand explanation of various mineral and chemical imbalances. When Tracey's chemical imbalance became severe she would feel sick. Now that she has this problem under control with supplements and diet she is feeling much better.

Dr. Books would get Toronto's and Tracey's bodies into alignment, relieve their aches and pains, and send them back to work where they would once again get out of alignment.

Dr. Books did a lot of counseling concerning emotions with both of them, as well as chiropractic and "Books Neural Therapy™" treatments. A screen writer, who also happened to be Toronto's meditation teacher, noticed Toronto's improvements during his sessions in Texas. About half way through a two-week series of treatments, Toronto called his meditation teacher to explain why he would be missing some classes. The writer/teacher listened to the changes in his voice and said, "Whatever she's doing, stay there. She's accomplished more with you in a week than I've been able to do in two years."

Toronto and Tracey were so impressed by, and grateful for, the relief they were receiving from Dr. Books' treatments that they set up a meeting in Los Angeles with several friends from the movie industry. Dr. Books treated their friends one after the other all day long. They all felt better after the treatments.

The many improvements in their lives seemed like a miracle to Toronto, Tracey and to me.

21

Do you have a friend who is DYSLEXIC and sometimes gets CONFUSED? BETH was.

Beth is a sweet, fun-loving, happy seven-year-old girl who likes being outdoors, playing with bugs, and riding her bike. However, Beth's teachers noticed that she was academically challenged and gave her extra time and help to get her work done. She had trouble paying attention (asking people to repeat what they said), and was often distracted from her schoolwork. It was hard for her to concentrate, follow instructions—especially if several were given at one time, complete assignments or tasks, and remember what she read. Concepts were difficult for her. She also reversed her numbers and letters, confused left and right, and got lost easily. It was hard for her to print and get the direction of the numbers correct. She had difficulty telling a story. Many of these were symptoms of **dyslexia**. The school had tested her for possible learning problems.

Physically, Beth had trouble with motor coordination, although she was good at running and standing on the balance beam. But when asked to tap her feet and make circles with her fingers at the same time, she was unable to do so.

Her goal for treatments was that she could get her homework done without outside help, and that she could think things through in an organized fashion. One of her mother's goals was that Beth's stories would have a beginning, middle, and an end. After her treatments Beth was able to do two things at one time, such as clapping her hands and moving her feet at the same time.

Another significant improvement was catching a ball with both hands. Before her treatments, out of five tries she was only able to catch the ball two times; after the treatments she caught the ball all five times. This was a big improvement in eye-hand coordination. Throwing a ball at a target improved from three hits to four hits. On the response speed test she was able to see the movement and respond to it much quicker. Out of seven tries she improved her median score from six to eleven points.

In drawing a line through a one-sixteenth of an inch path she went out of the lines twice before treatment; after treatment she was able to stay within the lines. Another eye-hand coordination test was sorting cards into stacks of red cards and blue cards. Before treatments she was only able to sort nine cards in fifteen seconds. After being treated she was able to sort twenty-seven cards in fifteen seconds. At the second-grade level it is important to see the improvement in gross and fine motor skills.

There was a lot of change in her handwriting. Her letters were more legible, even for a second grader. In young children we often see the improvement in their gross and fine motor skills first. Some need a little tutoring, or it takes a few months to catch up academically to their grade level. The important difference is that after treatments they do not have to continue all through school lagging behind their peers scholastically.

22

Do you know a young person who is DYSLEXIC and ABUSED DRUGS? JOSHUA did.

Joshua was forty-nine when he joined our summer program.

Joshua was the middle child in a family of three children. His mother was on thyroid medication during her pregnancy with him. She had false labor pains for four months. Finally, the doctor induced labor and used forceps to deliver Joshua. His parents were both supportive and good role models. But Joshua had learning disabilities.

When he was about five he had a bad fall and landed on the back of his head. This incident more than likely contributed to many of his problems, at least his parents noticed a difference in him after the fall—his intelligence decreased.

Joshua started school in Venezuela, where his father worked. When his family returned to California he had to repeat first grade in a school in Santa Ana, and was placed in remedial reading classes throughout his school years. He reports emphatically that he never liked school. Mathematics, concentration, reading, spelling, and memorizing were difficult for him, so he avoided them as much as he could. Actually, he just quit trying. Also, he preferred using his left hand but was forced to use his right.

The doctors prescribed Ritalin when he was a child, which did not help him.

As a teenager he was diagnosed as **dyslexic**. His resulting low self-esteem led to the abuse of drugs, which caused more stress. He also had a tendency toward falls, accidents, and suffered from emotional traumas and restless sleep. When things did not go well he would grind his teeth.

Joshua related well to animals; he loved the outdoors. As a youth he was labeled a "bum" because he did not like to stay in one place very long. When he became an adult he loved to travel. He is very outgoing, good with people, and finds it easy to make new friends. As an adult he suffered pain and stiffness in his joints, especially his knees and shoulder. He had tried both acupuncture and kinesiology.

An opportunity to be treated by Dr. Books through a scholarship sounded like a good opportunity to find out if he could improve his life, build his self-confidence and self-esteem, and discover what he wanted to do with his life. He set goals to become a better reader, writer, and improve his memory skills.

As his treatments under Dr. Books progressed he did become a better reader. The timing of the Summer 2001 project coincided with the popularity of the new Harry Potter book. Dr. Books found that she could entice kids into reading about the magical Harry Potter. Joshua, our forty-nine-year old, was no exception. He went out and bought all the Harry Potter books, as well as other well-known classics. His sister reported finding him in his room, reading, rather than out partying.

Joshua's spelling improved, he was writing more fluidly, his thought processes were more organized, and he felt less pain, all pleasant changes. Because he was an older man he was able to recognize the changes in himself and became capable of expressing his feelings regarding the improvements.

When his treatments were completed, Joshua enrolled at Santa Barbara City College. However, he owned a business in another country and was called to return there to take responsibility for the business. He felt that he was improved enough to leave the United States and continue his life.

Years later, his improvements are still holding. His sister and his entire family are thrilled. Books Neural Therapy ™ isn't limited just to children; Dr. Books likes to say it's for "kids of all ages".

23

Do you know a child who was diagnosed with ASPERGERS SYNDROME or AUTISM And was treated with RITALIN or PROZAC? POOR GEORGE was.

George had a difficult birth. After fourteen hours of labor the doctors did a C-section. A difficult birth is often hard on a child. Beginning when he was about four months old, George had a lot of earaches. From eighteen months until he was three or four years old he would bang his head on the wall. During early childhood George had asthma, allergies, rashes, problems with digestion, and with sleeping. He had frequent temper tantrums, including biting. Once he fell and broke his collarbone. Sometimes he would cry for no apparent reason, other times he would hug and kiss people.

Sitting still and concentrating was a problem. Socializing was also difficult, because he would sometimes invade other people's space, and tell lies on them. Teachers gave George an extra year in preschool hoping it would help him develop social and academic skills. When he was in kindergarten George tested high with intelligence and problem solving at a nonverbal level. Although his processing speed was slow, his error rate was low. His attention span was inconsistent. His test scores put him below the tenth percentile in most areas. He was above average in verbal reasoning but below average in other areas. The family (grandfather, and one uncle) had some history of reading difficulties and emotional dysfunction. His grandfather and uncle were bipolar.

George's gross and fine motor skills were poor. His movements showed mild developmental delays, and he confused right and left. He had a balance problem, so learning to ride a bike without training wheels was impossible. Throwing or batting a ball, tying his shoes, and doing other physical things that were easy for other children his age, were very difficult and frustrating for George. Sometimes he would put great effort into the task at hand, using his left hand to help the right, moving his tongue and mouth to aid in the muscular strain.

On some occasions he would miss or misunderstand instructions. Sometimes he was slow at processing information. Other times he would try very hard to be correct. When he was off in his own thoughts he hated to be disturbed. When George got involved in a task he would get lost in it and refuse to change to another subject or activity. On occasion he would get so overwhelmed when asked to change from one task to another, that he would become angry and contentious.

According to reports from his teacher, school principal, parents, and a testing psychologist, George, at seven years of age (first grade), was a very complicated child. At times he was very loving, even hugging his teachers and friends, eager to get attention. Other times he was belligerent toward his parents, teachers, and other children.

George enjoyed science, art, and music. The kids called him the "Science Guy". He had a vivid imagination and original ideas. He had a good sense of humor and enjoyed sports. Despite these good qualities George was having trouble in class. Putting together words and sentences was difficult. Writing was slow and the letters poorly formed. Math concepts were incomprehensible to him. When he was asked to focus on the class work he would sometimes lose his temper. On other occasions he would blurt out inappropriate words and, some days, he would even hit other children.

Frequent bouts of sadness, worry, fearfulness, temper outbursts, complaints of tiredness, tummy aches, and not feeling well, were some of his problems on school mornings. When he was too frustrated he would blurt out, "I'll just kill myself".

George was sent to a Ph.D. for a neuropsychological evaluation. The summary was: "His inattention and difficulty focusing are enough to impair both his academic and social functioning. He meets the criteria for Attention Deficit Disorder." His first-grade file shows repeated trips to the principal's office for behavior problems. Almost every day he would have a "time out" from class.

By spring George's behavior was deteriorating even more. He was defiant, needy, and erratic. Shortly after his eighth birthday he was diagnosed with **Aspergers Syndrome** and **ADD**. After considerable testing, one of the medical doctors started him on **Ritalin**, but the drug did not provide any improvement in his behavior, social skills, or schoolwork. The medical doctors also tried him on **Prozac**, which took the edge off of his behavior a tiny bit. Unfortunately his behavior worsened when his allergies were greatest. Doctors at UCLA's neuropsychiatric hospital noted some neurological disorders and diagnosed him as **autistic**. When he became excited, he would shake his head and flap his hands.

Sometimes he laughed or cried for no reason, said things out of context, and would grind his teeth at night. The tests given by other professionals delineated his problems, but did not provide much improvement in his life. Even at age eight, he still could not ride a two-wheel bicycle because he had balance problems. Staying focused on schoolwork was hard for him to deal with.

George was eight years old when he entered our summer program at the end of his first grade. His goal was to have less stress with schoolwork, to be less disruptive, and to have more confidence. After only eighteen treatments from Dr. Books, using "Books Neural Therapy™", his reading score improved from the 39th percentile to the 55th percentile. His math improved from the 13th to 19th percentile. We used the "Wide Range Achievement Test" before and after treatments to compare scholastic results.

To test his gross and fine motor skills we used the "Bruininks-Oseretsky" test of motor proficiency. He moved from the 14th to the 30th percentile. Before treatments he could only walk two steps, heel to toe, before stepping off the balance beam (the beam was only two inches off the floor), but he did four steps in a row after treatments. Before treatments he was not able to stand on one leg on the balance beam long enough to time him, he was just on and off. After Dr. Books' treatments he stood on one leg for eight seconds. Throwing a ball at a target improved from two hits to four hits after treatments.

Checking with his parents in March of the following year, seven months after his treatments, his father was very happy that now "his son could ride a two-wheeler without help". Before Dr. Books worked with him, he had a lot of trouble trying to handle a basketball. "Now he can dribble the ball and play basketball." Once his physical body and neurological pathways were gently and precisely adjusted and balanced, his academic skills, social skills, motor skills, balance, and behavior improved dramatically. "The teachers do not have trouble with his behavior in school as they did in prior grades. He is now reading ahead of his class and is up with his class in math." All these improvements in such a short time seemed like a miracle to me, and to his parents.

* George is number 8 in the California Research Project 2001 Summer Group

24

Did you have an ACCIDENT that left you DISORIENTED? WALLY did.

Dr. Books called me one morning to tell me that she had a patient coming from Texas with his mother for a week, "Could you please keep them at your house and test him before and after treatments?" Of course I said yes. I welcomed this lovely mother and handsome young man from Texas. Wally was a college football player; how he was able to come to Solvang is a story.

In 2001 Dr. Books had a doctor friend in Michigan do statistical work for us. I would send him the pre- and post-test results of our spring and summer groups and he would put them into charts and graphs and return them via computer. This doctor knew another doctor who worked with students in the school truancy department. This particular year they received a grant to cover the charges for four of these young people to receive treatments from Dr. Books.

Dr. Books went to Michigan during Easter vacation. Three teenage boys and one young lady showed up. Dr. Books worked on them, three sessions a day for five days, a total of fifteen treatments each. Wally's aunt was the attorney for the program. She had a knee problem, which Dr. Books offered to treat. Miraculously, her knee was 100 percent better after one treatment. The physician in charge informed her about the success of the treatments on the students. She was so impressed that she called her sister in Texas, and told her, "You have to get Wally to see Dr. Books. She did more for these boys in one week than we could do in two years."

As a college football player, Wally was muscular and well coordinated. (He had long black hair that stood out all over. When Dr. Books began working on his head she asked his mother to braid his hair so that she could feel his skull.) After receiving an injury to his shoulders during training, he became disoriented on the football field and didn't know where he was.

When Wally and his mother arrived, I tested him before the treatments began. In the Bruininks-Oseretsky test of Motor Proficiency, Wally reached a score of 88. Then Dr. Books gave him his first treatments. I was out of town when Wally finished his first sessions so I didn't get to test him right after the treatments.

He went to Virginia for a family gathering and something happened on the trip that knocked him out of balance again. He came back for a weekend in July. Dr. Books treated him and he was fine again, so I got to post-test him. His motor skills had improved so that he tested at 92. In the post motor skills test Wally's running speed and agility had improved by two points; his biggest improvement was in walking forward on the balance beam. His writing skills also improved.

His school recognized not only the physical improvements in Wally, but also an improvement in his attitude. His speed and accuracy on the field was noticeable to his trainer. Strange things happened in his reading score. It actually went down a couple of points, which can happen at the college level when the students encounter new and unfamiliar words. He misspelled three words in his second spelling test but re-testing resulted in a better score with familiar words.

In his Test Of Variables of Attention (T.O.V.A.), a visual continuous performance test for attention disorders, he improved.

After Dr. Books straightened out Wally's body and put it in balance he was an inch taller, from six-one to six-two, and six pounds lighter—from 256 pounds to 250 pounds. His walk was more even and Wally was better oriented to where he was.

Many times, patients and their parents are so private that they don't want anyone to know they are coming for treatments. We respect these patients' wishes in that regard. However, in Wally's case he and his mother were very open and glad to talk about the pain he was suffering and the severe headaches that had kept him from performing to the best of his ability. They were so grateful for the improvements made by Dr. Books' treatments, and to be able to stay at my home, that they gave permission to use their names. However, we cannot reveal the college he attended.

Wally's happy smile at the end of his treatments showed how much better he felt. His mother left a note that said, "Thank you, thank you, thank you, Mrs. Dotz. I pray that God blesses you always. You are a blessing. I know that your heart is running over with love. Thank you from Wally and Frances Smith." Because Wally went on to play professional football after college, we changed the family's names after all.

25

Have you tried EVERYTHING MONEY COULD BUY And it didn't help your child's READING ability very much? ANDREW'S family did.

A beautiful silver BMW convertible drove into my driveway one day. Out stepped an attractive, petite, young mother accompanied by a handsome little boy, Andrew, who ran across the lawn with rosy cheeks and a pleasant smile.

I had told Andrew's grandmother about Dr. Books' work on children with learning difficulties. Andrew, age ten, had been under all kinds of specialists and received every kind of help that money could buy, but nothing helped. He was in the fifth grade but, even with the help of a tutor, he could read only at the second-grade level. After completing Dr. Books' series of Books Neural Therapy™ treatments, in three months, he was up to the fourth-grade level.

In the questionnaire that Dr. Books has all patients fill out before beginning treatments, Andrew's mother indicated that, although he was good at memorizing, he had difficulty in reading, was slow at visual processing, and was hampered in learning Spanish, a required course at his school. Spelling was very difficult for him, math was a little easier. Her goal was that Andrew would be able to read fluently and with comprehension at grade level.

Since the doctors had diagnosed Andrew as **dyslexic**, his teachers often gave him extra time to do his schoolwork. (His mother's sister is also **dyslexic**.) Otherwise he was in good health and physically active—soccer, basketball, tennis, volleyball, golf, skiing, skateboarding, surfing, snow boarding—a very outgoing personality. He loves music and took guitar lessons. The youngest of three children, Andrew had a normal birth, crawled and walked at the normal age, lived under very little stress, and had parents who were good role models.

Before his treatments, his Bruininks-Oseretsky tests of gross and fine motor skills put him at the 50th percentile. After treatments were completed three months later, both his gross and fine motor skills had improved so much that he raised his score to the 99th percentile for a boy his age, an amazing improvement in so short a time!

Instead of writing down the page Andrew now wrote across the page and his work was much neater. His Wide Range Achievement Test reading score jumped from second to fourth grade level, which is from the 5th percentile for a child his age to the 27th percentile. In arithmetic he improved from the 21st to the 24th percentile.

After treatments Andrew had full control of his arms and legs, which he had not had before. The scale showed he had gained a pound in weight, from eighty-nine to ninety pounds and had gained almost an inch in height—partly due to natural growth; partly because his spine and body were now straightened.

We did the vision-screening version of the Test Of Variables of Attention (T.O.V.A.), a visual continuous performance test of Attention Deficit Hyperactive Disorder (ADHD). He improved from minus 5.76 to a minus 3.15—still in the minus range, but a great improvement. The normal range is -1.00 to +1.00. (Some doctors use this test to adjust the amount of **Ritalin** they prescribe.) The "correct" responses to the test improved from 622 to 633, and his "time" and "attention" responses also improved.

Seeing such a big improvement in his reading and motor skills in such a short time was like a miracle to his mother, grandmother, and me. Over the next four years his mother would occasionally contact Dr. Books to do a "tune up" on him.

26

Is SIXTY TOO OLD to be helped? JANICE was helped.

Attractive, petite, sixty-year-old Janice looked more like forty. She complained of attacks of chronic anxiety, and bouts of **dizziness** and **disorientation** while driving her car. As a little girl she had fallen out of a car. Although there appeared to be no outward injury, evidently she was injured internally. When Janice first came to Dr. Books she was tired, listless, and felt like her brain was in a fog.

School had been difficult for Janice. She had problems concentrating and memorizing what was required, yet she was very good at spelling and had good coordination. Because of her dedication and hard work, she was able to graduate from college with a teaching credential.

Janice likes to meet people one on one but would become stressed in large groups. She went from doctor to doctor seeking help and was given various treatments, including acupressure. Still, she was not satisfied with her condition.

After only two treatments with Dr. Books she was feeling better; after the fifth treatment she was able to drive her car from Monterrey, California, to Solvang—two hundred miles—by herself, without getting lost, which was an exciting experience for her and made her very happy. Her body was functioning with her, rather than against her.

Janice also suffered from digestive problems. The "gut" is considered a primitive brain often sending out stress signals before our real brain even registers what's going on. Dr. Books had to gently work to relax her colon and her entire digestive system so that the gut and brain could relax and communicate clearly instead of initiating anxiety and panic attacks.

The body is marvelously complicated with one system interdependent upon another. Stress to the structure and neurological systems can affect other organs and systems. Getting them all working together is quite an accomplishment.

Finding someone who can address several systems, instead of isolating just one, is another major achievement.

A year after her treatments with Dr. Books, Janice suffered a slight trauma and returned for a few treatments, until she felt fine again. Over the next few years she came to rely on Dr. Books' treatments for various health concerns. She also referred several family members and friends to Dr. Books.

27

Are you willing to GO THE EXTRA MILE for your children? Louis & Curt's parents did.

Thank God for mothers, fathers, and grandparents who are willing to go the extra mile to help their children be successful. There are many, many of them. The mother of Curt and Louis is one of them. She would get up early enough to get her two sons to Solvang by 7:30 A.M. (a thirty-five mile drive each way), to be treated by Dr. Books, and then return them to Santa Maria for school.

Curt, age sixteen, had been in special classes since second grade. His parents were hoping for any improvement in his learning difficulties. Brother Louis, fourteen, was in regular classes but wanted to ease the struggle he went through to do his best.

In his pre-treatment tests Curt, in tenth grade at the time, tested at the third grade level in reading and spelling and the fifth grade level in arithmetic. Twenty treatments later, over four months, Curt had improved to the sixth grade level in reading and the eighth grade level in arithmetic—a jump of three grade levels in four months for reading and math. However, he remained at the third grade level in spelling.

Dr. Books treated each boy with Books Neural Therapy™, starting with their feet, Achilles tendons, hips, pelvises, spines, and scapulas. Then she treated their necks, TMJ, jaws, cranial joints, and finally the sphenoid bones, and muscles around their eyes.

Louis had fewer kinks in his neurological system so he required fewer treatments. His body adjusted faster because he was younger and lighter in weight than his brother Curt. Louis, in the eighth grade, tested at the ninth grade level in reading, fifth grade in spelling, and tenth grade in arithmetic before his treatments. After twelve treatments over a four-month period, he improved to twelfth grade level in reading and arithmetic and sixth grade level in spelling.

The boys and their family were exceedingly grateful for the improvements in their lives. To me, as a former schoolteacher, it seemed like a miracle.

Several years later I was sitting in an airplane in Santa Barbara, waiting for take-off, when a lovely young lady, another passenger, came up to me and gave me a hug. It was an aunt of Curt and Louis. She had worked for us in our men's store when she was a teenager. She later opened her own men's store in Santa Maria and was now happily married and the mother of a young boy and girl.

When the plane reached flying level I was able to go back and visit with my friend's mom, who was Curt's and Louis's grandmother. Six members of the family—including Dad and Grandpa—were on a vacation to Washington D.C. to see the sights.

Their Grandmother brought me up to date on Louis and Curt. Both boys had graduated from high school. Curt was taking an apprentice program in construction at Alan Hancock College. (He started at cleaning, moved up to framing and was installing dry wall.) He had his own tools and was doing well. He still lived at home. Louis was also at Hancock College and would graduate after one more semester. He planned to continue his studies at San Diego State College. Louis's major was graphic arts. He was doing very well.

* Curt is number 7 in the California Research Project 2001 Spring Group

* Louis is number 8 in the California Research Project 2001 Spring Group

28

Has your friend gone from DEATH TO LIFE? DUDLEY did.

"Get your affairs in order. There's nothing more we can do for you," is what the doctors told Dudley. Dudley had been to more than twenty doctors throughout the year, who had prescribed various antibiotics and treated him in other ways for what they sometimes diagnosed as **Lyme disease**, yet he was getting progressively worse.

In July, when Dudley first got sick, his left side went numb, then his right side went numb, then his whole head went numb. He went to the hospital emergency room and they said he was having a **panic attack**. Dudley had been a big-rig truck driver for twenty-four years and had driven throughout all forty-eight continental United States. The next day, after visiting the emergency room, he drove 180 miles the wrong way, something he had never done before. As a result, he felt it was no longer safe for him to be driving a big moving van. At the end of August Dudley went to live with his parents, who were very supportive. Some days he felt so bad he would cry for four hours at a time.

After being diagnosed with **Lyme disease** Dudley tried to see a specialist. When the doctor's office found out that it was necessary for him to be on public assistance they escorted him out of the office. He was going to the hospital once a week with panic attacks. A physician at the hospital sent him to a psychologist who told him there was nothing wrong. After three or four weeks of this routine he still had **depression** and had received no help except to be put on several series of antibiotics.

At the beginning of January Dudley felt it was not Lyme disease but some type of metabolic or nutrition problem. Dudley was a triathlete for many years and entered races wherever his work took him. He had competed in more than thirty triathlons and five Ironman contests. So he was very aware of health and nutrition. He took himself off the antibiotics on his own and put himself on two thousand milligrams of calcium and a thousand milligrams of magnesium per day; the **depression** left, but he was still getting weaker.

Dudley prepared to die. He was too weak to hold a job. After four failed attempts he finally made it to his home in Austin, Texas. He planned to gather his personal belongings and return to his parent's home in Pennsylvania to await the end. He was at a nutrition store in Austin when a clerk told him about Dr. Books, and said that she had an instrument that could tell what was wrong with him.

Dr. Books received Dudley as a patient and listened to his problems. Then Dr. Books put Dudley on the QXCI/SCIO, a biofeedback assessment tool to get more definite information. (Over 28,000 of these machines are now in use worldwide.) This instrument will check for over nine thousand diseases, as well as nutritional, hormonal, and emotional stressors at the rate of 1/1000 of a second. Similar to a virus scan on a computer, it detects weaknesses such as viruses, nutritional deficiencies, allergies, and abnormalities by calculating the biological reactivity and resonance in a person's body. The Scientific Consciousness Interface System (SCIO) helps to access information from the unconscious and bring it to our awareness so it can be healed.

The machine listed many of Dudley's problems; pancreatic flukes; liver flukes; and parasites throughout his body were the worst. Dr. Books treated Dudley with Books Neural Therapy™, the QXCI/SCIO machine, the Ionic Cleansing Foot Bath, (the foot bath energizes the water to remove the toxic substances from the body via osmosis through the large pores of the feet, attracted by the highly-concentrated ion field in the water), and natural herbal remedies.

Dr. Books also took hair samples and sent the samples to the Analytical Research Labs, Inc., in Phoenix, Arizona, where they were tested for more than fifty different nutrient minerals, toxic metals, other minerals, and nutrient mineral ratios. When Dudley had panic attacks the doctors tried him on Paxil and Zoloft, which made him so sick he was suicidal. The hair test showed he had too much copper (among other imbalances) and needed to take zinc to balance out his system.

Dudley had no income and no place to live. Being on the road for two or three months at a time was hard on his family life. (The father of two grown children, he had been divorced for several years.) He stayed in a five-by-eight-foot enclosed motorcycle trailer behind a grocery store, basically homeless for a month and a half, in order to save money for his treatments. He ate healthy fresh foods. After ten treatments Dudley began to feel better.

Dudley's health continued to improve. He had a total of twenty-eight treatments. According to Dudley, "The energy Dr. Books channeled in to me with her 'hands on' treatments was incredible."

Dudley was so grateful to have a new chance at life he said, "I asked God, 'What do you want me to do?'" Dudley felt that he should help Dr. Books, so he started volunteering in her office, freeing Dr. Books to have more time for diagnoses and treatments. Dudley is kind and gentle with people; he feels that having been sick makes him more compassionate towards other people. He is good at putting people in and out of the twenty-two minute Detoxifying Ionic Cleansing Foot Bath for Dr. Books.

Dudley also feels that God has given him an ability to learn faster than he thought possible. He likes the study of nutrition and is quite knowledgeable, but wants to go for further training. He has taken special classes to become more proficient in the use of the QXCI/SCIO computer program. He wants to continue studying and become a naturopath so he can help more people, as Dr. Books does.

Dr. Books thinks so highly of Dudley's volunteer work that in July she invited him to be a full time member of the staff. He plans to continue studying under Dr. Books and take other classes and seminars.

Talking with Dudley a few weeks later, he said he was excited because his son was driving up from college in San Diego to visit him at the QXCI/SCIO Seminar in Santa Monica. When he had last seen his son at Christmas, he thought it would be for the last time, so he had given him some of his special things—like the special watch he used for timing his bike races. Dudley is so excited and thankful to have a new life ahead.

29

Did you know that Doctors' children can have LEARNING PROBLEMS also? These two medical doctors' sons did.

Dr. Nancy, Ph.D., and her husband Dr. Philip, M.D., are in practice in Santa Barbara. Dr. Philip is a psychiatrist, a physician who can prescribe medications; Dr. Nancy is a psychologist and provides counseling but no medications. Some patients of this distinguished looking couple, have addictive behaviors. One of the patients they had been treating for some time suddenly showed a big improvement. When they asked her what had changed in her life, she explained that she had been receiving treatments from Dr. Phyllis Books. The two doctors were so impressed by these changes that they called to set up an appointment with Dr. Books to meet for dinner so that they could find out why her treatments were so effective.

Over the years, from time to time, they met with Dr. Books at their favorite restaurant in Santa Barbara to discuss her procedures. Dr. Nancy treats some patients who have addictive behaviors with acupressure. Contrary to acupuncture, acupressure does not involve needles; rather, the doctor uses gentle digital pressure in a specified way on designated points on the body to relieve pain. Part of the treatment is to tape a bead on the part of the ear that is related to addictive desires. Dr. Nancy is trying to get that treatment more widely accepted because it helps to reduce people's cravings for addictive substances without the use of drugs. (This reminds me of how, years ago, some teachers would pull on a child's ear to get them to improve their behavior.)

With all the training the two doctors had, they were not able to help their own son, except to see that he received tutoring to get through school. When they met Dr. Books, their son Kyle—a charming, intelligent, tall, well-built, good-looking man, with a lovely wife and a good job—still had ADD.

As a child, as do most children with learning differences, Kyle put up with a lot of teasing and persecution all through school, because schoolwork was difficult for him. One day when he was eight years old he was riding his bike and when he turned a corner he went headfirst through a car's windshield and flew out the back window. After many surgeries he appeared fine; however, unknown to even his parents, he was now nearsighted in one eye and farsighted in the other. This condition—getting a different set of inputs to interpret—is very confusing to the brain. Dr. Books worked many combinations of therapies over his eyes and places where his accident impacted his body.

Kyle came in for double sessions since Dr. Books was only in town for a few days. After the second day, when he returned home to his wife, she said he "grew up." His voice was lower, his posture and carriage more grounded and centered.

Dr. Books likened this change to the Sleeping Beauty fairytale. It was as if a part of Kyle had been arrested at the age of eight, just as Sleeping Beauty went to sleep after choking on a bite of apple. When Prince Charming kissed her she coughed out the apple—and they lived happily ever after.

In Kyle's case, Dr. Books' treatments allowed Kyle to mature and grow up, a process that had slowed nearly to a stop when he had the accident. Now his inside matched his outside.

Kyle said, "I wish I'd had her help when I was a young child."

The doctors were so pleased by the improvements in their son that they began sending other patients to Dr. Books.

◆   ◆   ◆

One of my cousins, who was a medical doctor, Lieutenant Commander David, tall, handsome in his navy uniform, made an impressive entrance at family gatherings. After World War II he returned to his medical practice in Wauwatosa, Wisconsin. I remember him stopping in to visit us when his travels took him through Fond du Lac. He loved to reminisce with Mom about his boyhood summers spent with our family (before my time) when they lived on a farm that had cows, horses and a saw mill. Kent, one of Dr. David's three children, had mild to severe learning difficulties. The best they could do for him in those days was to put him in a boarding school for developmentally delayed children and adults so he could learn independent living skills. I felt very sorry for the family. It made me aware that learning problems are indiscriminate.

30

Do you know other doctors whose work is so unique it seems like a MIRACLE? DR. CHARLES KREBS from Australia is one.

Dr. Charles Krebs, a former Associate Professor of Marine Biology at the University of Maryland's St. Mary College, and his wife were returning from Germany on their way to Australia where they now lived. The Krebs had been in Germany where Dr. Krebs had taught his Learning Enhancement Acupressure Program (LEAP) at the Institute of Applied Kinesiology in Freiburg. They had stopped in Arizona to visit his sister and learned that Dr. Books was going to be at my house. Dr. Books had studied under him several years earlier and he wanted to meet with her again. So the Krebs changed their travel plans and came to Solvang, to my home. For a couple of days he and Dr. Books sat around my kitchen table, talking about their work with the brain, with kinesiology, and learning difficulties.

Dr. Krebs walked with a slight limp. He told us about the accident that caused it. Years before, he and his wife had been on holiday in Australia for a week of SCUBA diving with friends who were scientists and professional divers. Charles and two other divers made a deep dive, searching for a ship that had been wrecked in the 1800s off the spectacular Wilson's Promontory, one of Australia's most beautiful National Parks. Although the dive was technically perfect, Dr. Krebs suffered cerebral-spinal bends, with nitrogen bubbles forming in his brain and spinal cord. For the next ten days he and his two companions (who risked their lives trying to save Charles) lived in a deep decompression chamber at three hundred feet of pressure—something that had never before been done. It saved his life but severe damage had already been done. Charles came out of the decompression chamber a T-9 paraplegic, paralyzed from the waist down, and was in a wheelchair, never expected to walk again.

As he lay in his bed in the rehabilitation hospital, Charles first had to accept his condition. He *was* paralyzed from the waist down, whether this was "fair" or not! Just lying there, cursing his fate and wallowing in self-despair, was not going to get him walking again. So he used the tools he had to work with: a fairly photographic memory; a complete knowledge of the human nervous system giving him the ability to visualize the specific nerve pathway to each muscle in his paralyzed legs; years of martial arts training giving him the ability to move Chi with his mind. (Ch'i is a Universal Unseen Energy Force that exists in every physical thing, according to ancient Chinese practitioners and modern quantum physicists.) Working on muscle after muscle he re-activated most of his leg muscles so that he was able to walk out of the hospital after only six months—a true miracle to the neurologist who said, "I don't understand. You are one of the most neurologically damaged people in this ward!" However, today Dr. Krebs can walk quite well with only a slight limp.

Following this seemingly miraculous recovery, Charles began to investigate "alternative therapies" and came across Kinesiology—the study of how muscles connect to the energy systems of the body—and the Chinese acupuncture system. In an attempt to understand what happened to his body in the dive, Charles spent the next twelve years studying Eastern Energetic Sciences, as well as taking Kinesiology training. These studies led him to develop the Learning Enhancement Acupressure Program (LEAP).

As part of his work in Australia he ran a busy clinical practice treating children with Specific Learning Difficulties using his LEAP Program. More than 80 percent of these children improved in their reading, writing, spelling, math, and in social skills. Many went from being dosed with Ritalin, due to ADD or ADHD, to having good concentration and going off medication.

His technique is slightly different from that of Dr. Books. He has written a book about his injury and recovery, "*A Revolutionary Way of Thinking: From a near Fatal Accident to a New Science of Healing.*" It is full of great technical and practical information about learning and about the brain and how it works. The two doctors respect each other's ideas and abilities. Dr. Krebs has a new book entitled: *Nutrition for the Brain. Feeding Your Brain for Optimal Performance.*

Because this is a new field of research, doctors from different fields of medicine, seeking to improve their practices, get together to exchange ideas, discoveries, and problems. Once a year, some of them gather from all over the world and meet at the Annual International Conference of Kinesiology to discuss how they can help with cranial, neurological, physical and mental disorders, and learning disabilities.

We are so blessed to have so many talented people working and studying to find new ways to help their fellow human beings. Thanks and praise to God for inspiring them.

31

OTHER BOOKS WORTH READING

Corcoran, John, with Carlson, Carole C. *the teacher who couldn't read.* Colorado Springs, CO: Focus on the Family Publishing, 1994. The story of a boy who couldn't read, because of dyslexia, and other learning problems. How he used various tricks to get through school and college and become an illiterate teacher.

Dossey, Larry, M.D. *Healing Words, the Power of Prayer and the practice of Medicine.* San Francisco: Harper San Francisco, a Division of Harper Collins Publishers, 1993. Dr. Dossey has done extensive research on Prayer and its benefits to healing around the world and written several books on the subject.

Kaslow, Arthur L., M.D., and Miles, Richard B. *Freedom from Chronic Disease, A Drug Free Nutritional Program for Managing Your Health Problems.* Los Angeles, Jeremy P. Tarcher, Inc.,1979. Distributed by Houghton Mifflin Company, Boston, 1984. These men are pioneers in the relationship between food allergies and health and behavior problems. I saw a patient coming into their office in a wheelchair, suffering from Multiple Sclerosis. A few weeks later I saw her again and she was walking and doing fine after eliminating the foods she was allergic to.

Krebs, Dr. Charles, and Brown, Jenny. *A Revolutionary Way of Thinking: From a near fatal accident to a new science of healing.* Melbourne, Australia: Hill of Content, 1998. Dr. Krebs, with his wonderful academic background, has done much to standardize training in Brain Integration, Kinesiology, Acupressure, and more, in relationship to movement, memory, and learning.

Kroeger, Hanna. *GOD Helps Those Who Help Themselves.* Boulder, Colorado: Hanna Kroeger Publications, 1984. Hanna has written several books about God's gifts of herbs and God's rules for healthy living, and how we can use God's gifts in healing various diseases.

32

The Non Profit ASSISI FOUNDATION

The Assisi Foundation is a non-profit organization started by Dr. Phyllis Books and friends in 1994 in Irving, Texas. The federal 501 (c) 3 number is 75-2555282.

A branch was organized in Solvang, California, in 1998. The Foundation has conducted many fundraisers and received several grants. The board and officers are all volunteers. The funds raised are used to pay for testing and treatments for many, many patients. Donations may be sent to Assisi Foundation, c/o Books Family Health Center, 13740 Research Blvd. Suite M-1, Austin, Texas 78750.

ASSISI MISSION STATEMENT

The Mission of the Assisi Foundation is to enhance the lifelong learning capabilities by promoting a natural, gentle, non-drug treatment for resolving many common learning and behavioral problems.

A generous grant from the Schlinger Foundation made the California Research Project 2001 possible. We would love to do more projects like that.

Jail Population

Statistics vary indicating that any where from 60% to 90% of the people in jail can not read well enough to hold a good job. Wouldn't it be great if we could cut those numbers in half by using Books Neural Therapy™ to adjust their bodies so they could be successful?

33

Can you help your children learn by playing games with them? Yes you can.

There are games you can play with your children that make learning fun: for reading, math, spelling or other things.

1. When our country was founded the most common **reader** in the schools was the Bible. Gather the family around and take turns reading, adult one verse, child one verse. Start with an easy book, such as the book of John. Then try a book from the Old Testament such as the Book of Proverbs. Go to the New Testament again and try Luke. Psalms is another pleasant, easy to read Old Testament book. Then try some more from the New Testament. By alternating, child, adult, the children can hear how to sound the words and how to read with expression. A fringe benefit of reading the Bible is that children learn manners, morals, and human relations. They find words of comfort and words of inspiration.

2. The square wooden **BLOCKS** that little kids play with to build pyramids can also be used to teach them the letters and make words. The first word you want to make for them is their name. Some children can grasp the letters by sight. Some children can be helped to learn the shape of the letters by tracing over the letter with their fingers. As you play with them you can teach them the names of the letters and the sounds of the letters. Some blocks have animal pictures on some sides and alphabet pictures on other sides. Teach them the names of the animals and then, "What kind of sound does the animal make?" Same with letters: teach them the name of the letters and then, "What kind of sound does the letter make?" It can be fun if you include lots of laughter. Notice when the child is tired of the game and change to something else. Little children have short

attention spans. They learn quickly and forget quickly. Don't make it a chore. Let them know they are loved regardless of the outcome.

3. The alphabet song is the easiest tool for helping children learn alphabetical order. It was used in Europe generations ago. There is an old melody for it, but you might want to make up your own tune or rhythm.

ABCDEFG,
HIJKLMNOP,
QRSTU&V,
WX&Y&Z,
Now I've said my ABC's,
Tell me what you think of me.

4. The game of **SCRABBLE®** is the best for spelling. It's a game the whole family can play. The little wooden letters are easy to handle and are very durable. You may want to keep a dictionary handy for Scrabble®. The game makes an excellent Birthday or Christmas gift.

5. For basic **math** facts an easy game is this: Take an old standard (or bridge) deck of cards and set aside the face cards to begin. Show the child the ace is a one. The two has two hearts or diamonds, or spades or clubs. Then point out the three. Count the figures, then continue up to ten. Shuffle the cards and as you turn up the numbers ask the child to identify them. If they get it right it goes in their stack if they get it wrong it goes in the dealers stack. Make a happy smile or compliment when they get it right. Go thru the dealers stack again until they get them all right. After the children can recognize the numbers start putting them together in combinations for addition. At first slowly, give them time to see and add the spots. Gradually, by repeating the combinations, they will get to learn them by heart and by sight without counting them out. After they know their addition facts start with the subtraction facts. Then follow with the multiplication facts and the division.

Make it fun. Keep it short. Just a little at a time. The key is to repeat and repeat. Don't expect them to get them all right at first. Praise them for the ones they do get right. The attention span is different for each child, so don't keep them at it too long when they are little. As they grow older, you can also have them recite the multiplication tables as they are driving in the car on a long drive, not in heavy traffic. After they know the facts to ten, teach them the Jack has a value of eleven, the Queen twelve and the King thirteen. Then do the addition, subtraction, multiplication and division facts with those cards added to the deck. As the children develop their skills, games such as Fish, Concentration, Rummy, Canasta and Cribbage can challenge them. Let them keep score.

6. The **MONOPOLY®** game is a good one for teaching money values as children get a little older. Just remember to keep it fun. No cheating in any games.

7. When my son Richard was two years old I was watching a Roy Rogers Show on TV one day, when Roy was having Trigger, his horse, do math problems and giving the answer by tapping his hoof on the floor the correct number of times. I thought, "If he can teach a horse to count I can teach my two year old." So I said, "Richard, say, 'two'. Whenever I ask you a question say, 'two'. How old are you? Richard would say, 'two'. How much is one and one? Richard would say, 'two'. How much is 100 subtract 98? Richard would say, 'two'. What is the square root of 4? Richard would say, 'two'." I had a lot of fun saying, "See, my two year old can do square roots." When Richard went on to college he chose mathematics as his major.

8. Another game that can be fun is "**Detective**". Food and beverage detective, that is. The object of the game is to detect how food and beverages affect you or your child. You take a notebook or piece of paper and draw a line down the middle of the page. On the left side of the page you write down the date and everything you eat or drink that day. On the right side of the page you write how you felt afterwards. Did you feel stuffed and tired? Did you feel energized and wanting to move around? Did you have trouble staying awake during the day? Did you have trouble sleeping at night? Did you feel angry or irritable? What we put into our bodies effects how we feel and act.

Read the labels and see how much sugar they are feeding you. They have many different names for sweets, such as sucrose, fructose, cane juice, honey, corn syrup and others.

According to my friend Caro Stinson, R.D., Nutrition Services Supervisor, the extra large 64 oz. drink of carbonated beverage, cola, without caffeine contains 207.88 grams of sugar equal to about 50 teaspoons of sugar. The smaller 16 oz. bottle of carbonated beverage contains 64.93 grams of sugar equals about 16 teaspoons of sugar. The 12 oz. can of cola without caffeine contains 38.93 grams of sugar which equals about 9 teaspoons of sugar. Her figures are taken from the USDA Agricultural Research Service Nutrient Data Laboratory. Different brands or different kinds of soft drinks have differing amounts of sugar, but it varies by only a few teaspoons or grams. You can go to their

website http://www.nal.usda.gov/fnic/foodcomp/search/help.html for more information. (One teaspoon equals 4.2 grams of sugar.) Is it any wonder that young people
today are suffering from so much diabetes, tooth decay, and obesity, when they drink so
much soda and have so many sweeteners added to their foods?

One of my nephews drank mostly soda as a child and almost no milk. By age
25 he lost all his teeth and has to use false teeth the rest of his life. Visiting with a
friend the other day, she was telling me her 26 year old grandson needs $6,000.
worth of dental work. She is frustrated because she tried telling him not to drink
so much soda when he was younger. He wouldn't listen and now he is suffering.

God gave human beings a free will. You can choose what you put into your
body. The consequences are up to you.

9. **"Hide the Thimble"** is a game that is older than I am. If you don't have a
thimble in the house another small object will do. Any group from two or more
can play. While the rest of the group leaves the room the leader gets to hide the
thimble. It must be hid in plain sight. It cannot be inside another object where it
can't be seen.

When the leader is ready the others return to the room and start searching for
the thimble. If the search is lasting too long the leader may give clues. If someone
is moving closer to the object the leader may say, "You are getting warmer". If
someone is very close the leader may say, "You are getting hotter." The person
who finds the thimble first gets to be the next leader. This is a good game for
improving observation skills.

10. Another old game is, **"I Spy"**. The leader chooses an object to hold in his
or her mind that can be seen by every one in the room. The leader says, "I see
something _____." and names the color of the object. The other people are
called on in turn and say, "Is it _____?" and name an object that contains the
color mentioned. The first person to guess the right object gets to be the next
leader. This game helps with color identification.

Children need to exercise their eyes by moving them around to look at different directions and different distances, just as they need to exercise their bodies by
moving them around.

The hard part today is to turn off the TV, the computer and the radio, so the
children can concentrate on the game or on their homework. Check on how

much violence your children are learning from their video games. Are they learning to use their head to keep score?

Our children are only with us a few short years. They grow up and move out into the world. Spend time with them while you have them. The words they hear spoken at home are the words they will repeat when they are elsewhere.

Index

978-0-595-40915-0
0-595-40915-6